CONQUER TYPE 2 DIABETES

How a Fat, Middle-Aged Man Lost

31kg and Reversed His

Type 2 Diabetes

For Tracie, who knows everything there is to know about food.

CONQUER TYPE 2 DIABETES

HOW A FAT, MIDDLE-AGED MAN LOST
31KG AND REVERSED HIS
TYPE 2 DIABETES

Richard Shaw

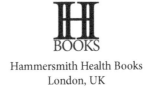

Hammersmith Health Books
London, UK

First published in 2019 by Hammersmith Health Books – an imprint of Hammersmith Books Limited

4/4A Bloomsbury Square, London WC1A 2RP, UK

www.hammersmithbooks.co.uk

Many of the recipes in this book feature shellfish and seafood. Please buy shellfish and seafood responsibly from sustainable sources. The Marine Conservation Society's Good Fish Guide is designed to help consumers; members of the fishing industry and retailers make the right sustainable seafood choices. Look for the blue MSC label on sustainable shellfish and seafood in shops and restaurants.

British Library Cataloguing in Publication Data: A CIP record of this book is available from the British Library.

ISBN (print edition): 978-1-78161-159-3
ISBN (ebook): 978-1-78161-160-9

Commissioning editor: Georgina Bentliff
Edited by: Dan Hurst
Designed and typeset by: Perrin Davis and Bespoke Publishing Ltd.
Cover design by: Jason Anscomb
Indexed by: Perrin Davis and Hammersmith Books
Production: Helen Whitehorn of Path Projects Ltd
Printed and bound by: TJ International, Cornwall, UK

www.conquertype2diabetes.com

Contents

CONQUER
’kɒŋk’ə

verb

Middle English from Old French *conquerre*, based on
the Latin *conquirere* (gain, win) from *con-* (expressing
completion) + *quaerere* (seek).

—*To overcome or take control of by force, defeat, beat,
vanquish, triumph over, be victorious over, mean to get the
better of, implies gaining mastery of.*

FOREWORD

Richard Shaw should be applauded for achieving what most people, including doctors, believe to be impossible: reversing type 2 diabetes.

In his book *Conquer Type 2 Diabetes*, Richard shows with clarity and in detail how this can be achieved. It is clear that it requires motivation, determination, and willpower, which Richard clearly has in spades. Through his remarkable weight loss, achieved by virtue of a low-carbohydrate diet and a short-term reduced-calorie approach, Richard completely reversed his diabetes in just a few months, proven through blood test results. So after years of over-indulgence and little exercise (by his own admission), Richard finally grasped the nettle and has now emerged as a healthier, fitter version of himself. He's now free of the risks of type 2 diabetes complications, which cause so much misery and cost and are, sadly, so prevalent in today's society.

Richard has proven that the answers to lifestyle diseases are not to be found in boxes and boxes of pills; instead, the answers lie in making lifestyle changes—most importantly those related to diet, with some exercise thrown in for good measure. And if you're a foodie, like Richard, you can still enjoy gourmet food on the diet he followed.

As a GP working in the NHS, I'll be using Richard's example—anonymised, and with his permission, of course—to show patients who have diabetes and really want to make changes and improve their health (and even those who don't) that it *is* possible, in many cases, to take control of their health and conquer type 2 diabetes.

—Dr Charlotte Mendes da Costa MRCGP MFHom

September 2018

ABOUT THIS BOOK

This book is a personal account of my battle with type 2 diabetes. There's an extended introduction that chronicles my journey through the diagnosis and an action plan that explains what I did to banish this disease and come off medications.

There's a short section about a light exercise regime that happened towards the end of the programme. And the last section is a collection of low-carb, low-sugar recipes that I hope might be useful.

Some of the recipes are incredibly simple and others are a little more involved, but all are within reach of an experienced domestic cook. I wanted to eat food that I enjoyed so I'm not ashamed to admit that some of the recipes are more elaborate than you might find elsewhere, but they worked for me.

I owe a great debt of thanks to the Kitchen Guru, Tracie Dudley Craig, one of my closest friends and a wonderfully talented chef, who has immeasurably improved the recipes and even come up with several of her own. You can follow her online at @tracie_dudley_craig.

If you're only interested in how this is done you can skip the next few pages and jump straight to the section headed The Plan (*see page 35*) but…

...BEFORE YOU GO ANY FURTHER

I wrote this book as a record of what I did to overcome this disease. But it is different for everyone and I'm not a healthcare professional, nor am I qualified to give medical advice. There can be some very significant risks associated with changing your diet and for some people these risks can be far greater than the original diagnosis itself. What worked for me may not work for you. Despite the fact that it's called the same thing, your medications may be different and your outcomes may be radically different from mine.

A type 2 diagnosis disguises a huge range of complications and underlying causes and as I started to understand a little more about this disease and talked to other people about their condition it became ever-more obvious that there is no one-stop shop that's right for everyone.

Before you do anything to challenge your diagnosis you must talk to your doctor or a professional dietitian or nutritionist and stay in touch with them throughout the process. Nothing in this book is right for children, adolescents, the elderly, those taking insulin, or pregnant women or those planning pregnancy, women who are breastfeeding, people in poor mental health or with other significant medical conditions, or people with type 1 diabetes or those with a very long-standing type 2 diagnosis. Trust me: I'm not a doctor.

Where I can offer some advice is on food, not only because I love to cook but also because I've faced down my own type 2 diabetes by radically changing my eating habits. Food has played an enormous part in both my professional and private life. I was trained at one of London's leading cookery schools. I've made food programmes for TV in both the UK and the USA, I've helped publish cookbooks and I even appeared on *Masterchef*. And in tackling this disease, I've wrestled with the complicated psychological hold that food has over us. And the good news is that, although I've dramatically changed my diet, my love affair with food endures, it is no longer toxic and I enjoy healthy, nutritious and delicious food that I know is nourishing my body.

I was inspired to do this after reading about the work of a remarkable team of scientists in Newcastle and Glasgow. This book has no formal relationship with their work, the Diabetes Remission Clinical Trial (DiRECT[1]) funded by Diabetes UK[2] into primary care-led weight management for remission of type 2 diabetes. But their findings inspired me in many ways, not least because they gave me the confidence to understand that something can be done about type 2 diabetes, that for many people it is reversible and that it is possible in many cases to both eradicate this disease and come off and stay off medications.

There are no guarantees in this process. Life is unpredictable. But a revolution is coming in our understanding of type 2 diabetes and the hundreds of millions of people worldwide who have this disease are arguably being short-changed by a poor understanding of the possibility of remission, by a long-standing dependence on conventional medicine and by decades of ineffective and counterproductive dietary advice.

Welcome to the diabetes revolution. And good luck in your journey.

—Richard
conquertype2diabetes.com

---

1 http://www.directclinicaltrial.org.uk
2 https://www.diabetes.org.uk

INTRODUCTION

When I started out on this journey I was a fat, 54-year-old man who did no exercise within five years of my diagnosis. And when I first raised the subject of reversing my diabetes, the idea was met with a degree of scepticism. In this respect I was unlucky. I've since come across many people who understand how this works, but when I started out I was told that it would both take tremendous willpower and that the likelihood of success was pretty low. Someone told me they had a book somewhere on the subject and that they'd send it to me. It never arrived, so I wrote my own.

A dietitian I discussed my diagnosis with told me that I'd probably never be free of diabetes and that there was a strong chance that I'd be on medications for the rest of my life. Without a big lifestyle change, I was told that my condition could become insulin-dependent. And perhaps the biggest obstacle to believing this could work was that I struggled to find anyone who had managed to overcome the disease by changing their diet.

In the last few years the idea of reversing type 2 diabetes has become a worldwide movement. Many thousands of people have done it, and the good news is spreading. There are some extraordinarily talented researchers working in this field and some great examples of ambitious early-stage public health interventions[3], but the real energy for change is coming from patients themselves—people who are successfully challenging their diagnosis and sharing their experiences with others.

By the time I had finished writing this book, both public and medical opinion was shifting a little. As I completed the weight loss and waited for the results of my blood tests, vanity got the better of me, and I posted a few before-and-after pictures of me on an online discussion forum. Within a few hours hundreds of people from across the world had responded with questions, encouragement and enthusiasm, many with their own stories to tell. And by the end of the week, the responses were in the thousands.

Many people were struggling with their diagnosis, angry at a system that was just too slow to keep up with the advances in medical science that held out the very real prospect of remission. One writer was particularly forthright. His views echoed the opinions of hundreds of others as he said,

> I'd like to take your pictures and cram them in the face of every arrogant and willingly ignorant medical professional who states that "diabetes is a progressive disease and will only get worse over time" as they continue to send people to their graves because of their hubris.

Rather more robust than I would have been, perhaps, but I got his drift, and a small part of me felt the same way.

I'm part of the self-diagnosis generation. The Internet gives us access to new choices and fresh information, but not all of it is reliable.

---

3   https://www.england.nhs.uk/2016/03/nhsdpp/

Medical science gives us mixed messages about how to deal with the food issues surrounding type 2 diabetes, and public policy and medical advice are in direct conflict with many people's personal experience. Should we eat carbs or should we not? Should we go high protein or low protein? Should we cut the calories? Is fruit good or bad? Is it to be full-fat or dairy free? It's a confusing picture.

As I read about the subject, I came across a clinical trial where people had used a change in diet to restore their natural pancreatic and liver functions. I desperately wanted to see if I could do this for myself, but I had no idea how to do it. In particular I had no idea how to change my diet to lose enough weight to overcome diabetes.

Even the word *diet* is contested. It implies something temporary, and although this book documents a process that happens over a few short months, this really does need to be a long-term lifestyle change. There's no point going through all the challenges of weight loss simply to watch the numbers on the scales creep back up in the long term and have the symptoms return. And if the word diet puts you off altogether, don't worry; this isn't a particularly unorthodox regime. I'm not proposing that you should only ever eat plants or become a fruitarian or eat cabbage soup for weeks. My approach is far less radical. I like food too much and lack the self-discipline to do any of these things.

After weeks of thinking about it, I decided to become my own lab rat and attempt my own version of a weight-loss regime—not only to lose the visible body fat I was carrying, but also to reduce the internal fat that I assumed was compromising my internal organs. It worked for me. It may not work for everyone. But the benefits that will come from losing weight and getting fitter will be worthwhile, even if it doesn't banish the disease for everyone.

I had a salutary moment as I came to the end of the process. A colleague who had watched my progress over the months confided that she had a friend who had followed an almost identical regime and lost a similar amount of weight, but his condition hadn't improved. Despite a monumental effort, his blood scores remained stubbornly within the clinical range that defined him as diabetic. Sure, he had lost weight and was healthier as a result, but his underlying diagnosis hadn't changed.

It's a lottery. But I figured that if I didn't play I'd have no chance of winning. So I rolled the dice.

THE FOREVER MYTH

When the diagnosis first arrives it's a shock. Looking back, one short sentence on the UK's National Health Service website really brought home how much this disease would affect my life: "Diabetes is a lifelong condition that causes a person's blood sugar level to become too high."[4] It was the phrase "lifelong condition" that rattled me. At that time, as far as I was aware, there was no fix—I'd done this to myself, and there was nothing I could do about it.

When I was first diagnosed in early 2012, I entered a whole new world of tablets, tests and examinations. I'd walk home from the pharmacy with a large bag bursting with boxes of pills and struggle to find the space to store them. For several years these tablets became as much a part of my life as toothpaste and mouthwash (and took up a lot more space in the bathroom), and when they ran out I'd go back for another enormous supply.

If the medications were demoralising, the dietary advice was even more dispiriting. Since the 1980s, people with diabetes have been encouraged to eat a low-fat diet, including prodigious amounts of starchy carbohydrates. For decades, public health advice has encouraged us to believe that up to half our energy should come from

---

4   https://www.nhs.uk/conditions/diabetes/

carbohydrates, which typically means consuming 200g to 300g of carbs a day.

Many people now believe that this is quite wrong—that this can actually promote weight gain, lead to high blood glucose levels and encourage a dependence on medication that only increases over time, leading to sufferers being prescribed stronger and stronger doses as they get older. Arguably, much of the type 2 dietary advice over the last 30 years has at best promoted a medication-based maintenance regime and at worst compounded the problem for millions of people worldwide.

I had bought into the predictions that many websites were offering: the prognosis appeared to be very poor. I Googled the words "do most people with type 2 diabetes eventually need to take insulin by injection," and website after website told me that I would probably be injecting myself eventually. I started to study the eating advice online in search of help.

The UK's National Health Service tells us that "people with diabetes should try to eat a healthy balanced diet … and to include starchy foods at every meal." We're told in an online NHS article, "The Truth about Carbs," that "the Government's healthy eating advice, illustrated by the 'Eatwell Guide,' recommends that just over a third of your diet should be made up of starchy foods, such as potatoes, bread, rice and pasta."[5] The "Eatwell Guide" goes on to suggest we eat five portions of fruit and vegetables, drink lots of water and "try to go for lower-fat and lower-sugar products where possible, like 1 percent fat milk, reduced-fat cheese or plain low-fat yoghurt."[6]

My subsequent experience was that this advice, about both carbohydrates and low-fat foods, was complete hogwash. It simply doesn't work if what you really want to do is lose enough weight to challenge

5   https://www.nhs.uk/Livewell/loseweight/Pages/the-truth-about-carbs.aspx
6   https://www.nhs.uk/Livewell/Goodfood/Pages/the-eatwell-guide.aspx

the underlying cause of a type 2 diagnosis. Many others now agree, including some progressive doctors and nutritionists, diabetes charities, MPs (who have even been moved to write to the Prime Minister on the subject[7]) and, above all, patients themselves.

As I settled into my diagnosis, a familiar routine developed. Automated letters from my doctor arrived with a request that I come in for an annual check-up or attend an eye scan or join a quit-smoking clinic. Prescriptions were sent directly to the pharmacy, and I would be summoned when they were ready. My disease was being "managed" in the most efficient way possible: it was a way to keep me stable, not a plan to conquer my diagnosis. I have nothing but the greatest admiration for my own personal GP, who provided endlessly wise counsel and sage advice in the years I had a diabetic diagnosis. The staff at the surgery I attended were both patient and attentive and offered encouragement, and always put up with my sulky attitude with considerable grace.

Annual check-ups were focused on the key issues of blood pressure, glucose scores, eye tests, waistline measurements and, rather unexpectedly, foot health. Diabetes can cause complications through nerve damage—a condition known as *sensory diabetic neuropathy*. For many people this can damage the feet and legs, as wounds become infected and very difficult to treat. Diabetes can also affect the circulation in your legs and feet as a consequence of peripheral arterial disease.

I went into a three-year sulk. I started skipping the appointments and throwing away the letters. Anyway, I was heading for daily injections in due course, so why bother? In my heart I knew it was all my fault. I had brought this on myself, and I was paying the price for a lifetime of bad habits.

---

7   https://www.facebook.com/notes/nathan-gill-mep/i-have-written-to-the-prime-minister-about-diabetes/2122397704647236/

Not long after my diagnosis, one of my best friends, Warren, came to stay. One morning I heard a loud exclamation as he opened the bathroom cabinet. 'What the hell?' he said as he came face-to-face with a precarious tower of medications.

Warren has lived all his life in northern California. He goes to the gym regularly, eats incredibly healthy food and spends his spare time sweating through hot yoga sessions and downing wheatgrass shots. His tall, lean, muscled and perfectly proportioned body is testament to his disciplined, sun-kissed, organic, West Coast lifestyle. He's a pale, lithe, muscled health nut who dances till he drops twice a week and never skips his early morning stretches.

By contrast, I was an overweight, indolent, lumbering middle-aged man who avoided physical exercise at all costs. I ate treacle tart and chocolate bars in alarming quantities. I drank litres of fresh fruit juice each day and consumed recklessly large amounts of sugar. My cornflakes were smothered in golden syrup, and I could demolish a whole Battenberg in one sitting. We were each impressive in our own ways.

As I saw his reaction to the medications, I realised that I'd normalised my diagnosis and the tablets that came with it. I'd succumbed to the idea that this was a "lifelong condition" without ever stopping to question it, believing wholeheartedly that there was nothing I could do about it and excusing myself from the effort of trying.

I came across a study by Newcastle University's Magnetic Resonance Centre that saw some people reverse type 2 diabetes by following a strictly monitored clinical diet. Eleven people had attempted to reverse their diagnosis by drastically cutting their calories to just 600 a day for two months. The subjects' austere regime was made up of liquid diet-replacement shakes, plus a further 200 calories a day of non-starchy vegetables. They were matched to a control group and monitored over eight weeks. At the end of the trial, seven out of the original 11 volunteers were diabetes free. My world stood still for a moment as I absorbed the implications of what I had read. Perhaps the grim prediction that I was heading for daily insulin injections was just plain wrong?

Many people lose weight to change the way they look. They want to get rid of the visible fat that accumulates around their midriff or that gives them flabby arms or a double chin, but the key issue for many type 2 patients is that internal fat can compromise the vital functioning of the liver and pancreas. This fat needs to be banished for the body to be able to effectively re-start and regulate its own blood glucose.

Professor Roy Taylor of Newcastle University, who led the study, was quoted as saying:

> To have people free of diabetes after years with the condition is remarkable—and all because of an eight-week diet. While it has long been believed that someone with type 2 diabetes will always have the disease, and that it will steadily get worse, we have shown that we can reverse the condition.[8]

THE RELATIONSHIP BETWEEN BODY FAT AND TYPE 2 DIABETES

Body mass index (BMI), the measure of weight compared with height, has long been thought to be an indicator of diabetes risk. There's a commonly held belief that overweight people are at greater risk of type 2 diabetes than those with healthy BMIs. But according to research, 70 percent of severely obese people don't have diabetes[9] and there are some very slim people who do. So what's the truth?

---

8   http://www.ncl.ac.uk/press/articles/archive/2015/10/type2diabetes/
9   http://www.ncl.ac.uk/press/articles/archive/2016/03/
profroytaylordiabetesresearch/

Research suggests that a predisposition to adult onset diabetes actually depends on how well your body stores fat, and this is different for everybody. Many people are advised to shed the visible stomach fat that accumulates over years of bad eating habits, but it appears that for some people, diabetes can be triggered by the accumulation of internal fat that disrupts the liver and pancreatic functions—organs crucial for producing insulin and regulating blood sugar.

A research paper on the website of the scientific journal *Clinical Science*[10] refutes the view that type 2 diabetes is solely a result of obesity or being very overweight. Instead, it argues that once someone goes above his or her own "personal fat threshold," the body's ability to control blood sugar starts to deteriorate until it eventually malfunctions. Crucially, the evidence also suggests that for many people, this process is reversible. Reduce the internal fat, and the body can restore blood glucose levels and insulin production to normal.

Not all type 2 diagnoses are the same. There are people for whom this excess fat issue isn't relevant. Their diagnosis comes from other causes, such as old age, pregnancy or chronic illnesses. Diabetes can be caused by chronic pancreatitis, and monogenic diabetes can't be reversed using weight loss. And for people who have had a type 2 diagnosis for more than six years, the odds of reversing the disease are rather lower.

I began to wonder if my own diabetes was being caused by internal fat that was compromising my normal organ function. If I could lose the weight and purge the fat, if my pancreas spluttered back into life and if my liver function wasn't too damaged, then perhaps my insulin levels would stabilise and the diabetes would just go away? It was a lot of ifs but it sounded reasonable, and it was the only thing I had to go on.

---

10 http://www.ncl.ac.uk/media/wwwnclacuk/newcastlemagneticresonancecentre/files/PersonalFatThreshold_Paper.pdf

Professor Roy Taylor, who led the original Newcastle University study, has published a simple and elegant five-page advisory[11]. In it, he makes the point that while substantial weight loss must be achieved, the speed of the weight loss is less important than the actual drop in weight. A small line buried in the document caught my attention: "Any pattern which brings about substantial weight loss over a period of time will be effective," he announced. The all-important word here was "will". Not "may," but "will". This single word was the spur I needed. Suddenly, instead of being told this was a life-long condition, I had a choice. I had the opportunity to do something about my diabetes, and if it worked, it might have a long-term effect.

If any further proof was needed, the results of a new and wider trial were published in November 2017. This study saw 306 people recruited from 49 primary care practices in Scotland and the Tyneside region of England achieve astonishing results. The study involved withdrawing all anti-diabetic and anti-hypertensive drugs, a total diet replacement with an 825 to 850 kcal/day formula for three to five months, a stepped food reintroduction over a two- to eight-week period and structured support for long-term weight loss maintenance.

Those who lost the greatest amounts of weight were the most likely to be successful. A staggering 86 percent of people who lost 15kg (33 lb) or more put their type 2 diabetes into remission[12]. More than half the people who lost between 10kg to 15kg achieved remission. Overall remission was achieved in 46 percent of the participants. The headline messages from this study, summarised by Professor Mike Lean

11 http://www.ncl.ac.uk/media/wwwnclacuk/newcastlemagneticresonancecentre/files/2017%20Diabetes%20reversal%20info.pdf
12 http://www.ncl.ac.uk/media/wwwnclacuk/newcastlemagneticresonancecentre/files/DiRECT1yearResults.pdf http://www.ncl.ac.uk/media/wwwnclacuk/newcastlemagneticresonancecentre/files/DiRECT1yrPaperSupplementaryAppendix.pdf These files are of the final manuscripts as copyright prevents posting of the full Lancet paper itself.

MA MD FRCP, Professor of Human Nutrition at the University of Glasgow, are so revolutionary that they're worth reproducing in full (with permission, see page 145):

> *Type 2 diabetes is a hateful disease, gradually, silently damaging vital organs and bodily functions. It is especially serious and shortens life significantly in younger people (under age 70-75). It is almost always in people who are overweight. We have shown, in research funded by Diabetes UK, that type 2 diabetes is not necessarily permanent. It can often be reversed into remission (non-diabetic again, taking no anti-diabetes medications) by sustained substantial weight loss.*
>
> - *With substantial weight loss (over 15kg) almost 9 out of 10 can achieve a remission (no longer diabetic, non-diabetic HbA1c, taking no drugs for diabetes treatment).*
>
> - *With weight loss of 10kg to 15kg, still over half can achieve a remission.*
>
> - *These figures apply to people with type 2 diabetes for up to 6 years. With longer duration, remission is still possible but less likely.*
>
> - *For smaller people (e.g. body weight under 70kg), lesser weight losses may be successful.*
>
> - *We do not yet know how long a remission of type 2 diabetes will last, but the key is maintaining the weight loss, and possibly losing more weight at a later stage.*
>
> - *Achieving a remission is the best bet to prevent, or at least delay, the complications of diabetes, but we*

cannot guarantee that they will be avoided for all patients as other factors may apply (e.g. high blood pressure).[13]

A full summary of the groundbreaking DiRECT trial is available on-line[14]. There's a qualification here: the volunteers in this trial weren't representative of the whole diverse population of the UK. This may be important for future research, as there is compelling evidence that type 2 diabetes is more prevalent in different populations around the world[15].

Studies that focus on disparities in glycaemic control have often been contradictory and have been compromised by excessively broad population and ethnicity categories, small sample sizes, limited follow-up, inadequate adjustment for socioeconomic differences and variations in levels of access to (or use of) healthcare. A large nationwide observational study from the Swedish National Diabetes Register between 2002 and 2011 aimed to comprehensively map glycaemic control in a large diverse cohort of patients with type 2 diabetes[16]. Their results called for more individualised management and increased efforts from the medical system to eliminate inequalities. Many scientists believe that type 2 diabetes is a consequence of both genetic and environmental factors, and the full implications of this for different people from different backgrounds attempting to reverse their disease through diet will only be fully understood in the decades ahead.

Progress is achingly slow. Doctors are only gradually becoming aware of the advances in research from the DiRECT trials. A brief paragraph from the earlier Newcastle study declared, "It will take

---

13 http://www.directclinicaltrial.org.uk/Documents/Patient%20Info%20Website%20Feb%202018.pdf

14 http://www.directclinicaltrial.org.uk

15 Nazroo, JY (1997). The health of Britain's ethnic minorities: findings from a national survey. London. Policy Studies Institute at Nazroo, JY (1997). https://www.diabetes.org.uk/resources-s3/2017-11/diabetes-key-stats-guidelines-april2014.pdf

16 http://bmjopen.bmj.com/content/5/6/e007599

years for this new knowledge to become incorporated into textbooks and guidelines, so your doctor may be wary of information from the Internet. Therefore, here are some notes for you to take to your doctor."[17]

There is surely something terribly wrong here. It seems almost unbelievable that patients need to become their own primary advocates for the advances in treatment of one of the most widespread illnesses of our generation. The National Health Service in the UK, staffed by dedicated and committed people who work long hours in service of the nation's health and well-being, is one of the country's greatest national assets. It is an extraordinary institution, and we are enormously fortunate to have it. But the inability of the medical profession to change swiftly and respond decisively to this revolution in the treatment of type 2 diabetes is deeply discouraging for the millions of people who suffer from this disease, many of whom might just stay on medications for decades.

Despite how promising the early trials sounded, I knew that the clinical approach wasn't for me. There was no way I could restrict myself to such a small daily calorie limit; I didn't have the self-control. Plus, to do the diet properly, I needed to get hold of the same magic meal replacement shake used in the trial. Clinical-grade food replacement products can be surprisingly tricky to get hold of, and many need to be prescribed by a doctor. I considered buying generic alternatives and even tried a few over-the-counter products, but they were all horrible. Professor Taylor refers to his approach to diet as "vigorous," and after considering the options for a while, I decided that his hard-core approach was simply impossible.

I knew enough to be aware that a calorie-restricted diet alone was unlikely to be sustainable in the long term. And in truth, I doubted

---

17 http://www.ncl.ac.uk/media/wwwnclacuk/newcastlemagneticresonancecentre/files/2017%20Information%20for%20doctors.pdf

my willpower to keep with the programme. There were other things about the original trial that made me wince. I've always loved food—not just eating, but also cooking and sharing meals with friends. The blanket prohibitions on meat, fish, poultry, carbs, dairy, fruit and alcohol filled me with gloom. Then there were the recipes. The original Newcastle meal ideas consisted of eight vegetable soups, a single salad, a recipe for tomato sauce and a salsa. If I wasn't enjoying the food in front of me then I was sure to fail. I needed something slower, less brutal and much more achievable.

I decided that I could attack the weight over a much longer period: still fast, but not quite so fast. And if I couldn't get the meal replacement product, I'd do it my own way. So I cherry-picked. There were to be no shake substitutes. Soup was good, although I'd use my own recipes. No meat or dairy was unthinkable. Low-carb was OK. Smaller portions I could cope with, and for reasons that become clear later (*see page 49*), I knew that consuming fewer calories than normal was only likely to be temporary. No alcohol I could do, for a while. A plan started to emerge.

I called the surgery to see the diabetes nurse. She took the normal bloods, examined my feet and quite rightly told me I was overweight while we made small talk about the Christmas break and our plans for the year. I talked to her about changing my diet to get rid of diabetes; she nodded and smiled and gave me a poorly printed leaflet containing several recipes for soups and salads and a list of exercises. I growled and left.

A week later the results were in, and again, they were terrible. But by then I'd already decided that I was going to declare war on this illness, and I was going to do it my own way. Taking inspiration from the Newcastle study I was going to purge the internal fat in my body by completely ignoring the NHS advice about diet, particularly when it came to eating carbohydrates and low-fat foods.

There is a word of caution here. The plan I devised wasn't particularly scientific. It has a focus on low-carb foods, reduced calories for a short period, fewer sugars, increased water intake and some exercise, but it's a blunt set of rules. I didn't do daily blood scores with test strips and didn't measure my ketones. I don't generally calculate "net carbs". More scrupulous people will carefully balance fat intake against carb reduction and carefully compare glycaemic index (GI) numbers with glycaemic load scores and chart their results. But I simply took a deep breath, set myself a series of five very simple rules and ruthlessly stuck with them.

The results are proof that for many people, type 2 diabetes doesn't have to be a lifelong condition and that you can take a shot at reversing your diagnosis if you really want to.

I swear, if a slacker like me can try it, so can you.

THE DOUGHNUT MOMENT

I've never been disciplined in my eating. And it started early. At home my father baked vast Yorkshire puddings and served them with gravy as a comforting starter in the traditional Yorkshire manner. I spent my early years at university blowing my student grant by eating my way through all the restaurants and fish-and-chip bars that Hull (one of my favourite cities; it's on the northeast coast of the UK) had to offer.

Food dominated my social and, eventually, my professional life. I spent over 30 years living and playing well, and I had the waistline to prove it. My capacity for takeaway Indian food and deep-pan pizza was limitless. I had cabinets full of Mars bars and freezers full of ice cream on standby for lazy weekend afternoons. The weekly shopping trolley was loaded with croissants and cakes, rice and fresh pasta, and I was consuming at least a litre of fresh fruit juice every day, often more. I attended a prestigious London cooking school where we were ruthlessly drilled in the precise arts of classic pastry and fresh pasta making. I appeared on *Masterchef,* and a career in TV production producing food and travel programmes beckoned, which fuelled my interest in food even more.

I met a hugely talented chef, Tracie Dudley Craig, whom I promptly christened "the Kitchen Guru." I was delighted to find someone who liked eating almost as much as I did. We started travelling the world together with the singular aim of discovering a city through its food.

I ran away to Florida in early 2012. Travelling alone, I hired a car for two weeks to drive the coast road from Cape Canaveral to Key West. In the weeks leading up to the trip I'd been feeling listless and exhausted. My friends had told me that I needed a break and that I should turn off the phone and get some sun. Although undiagnosed at the time, I was already displaying some of the classic symptoms of type 2 diabetes. Despite dropping a little weight (recent unexplained weight loss is a classic symptom of type 2 diabetes) I was still vastly overweight.

Although the words were unknown to me at the time I was already experiencing polydipsia, polyuria and polyphagia—pretty words for excessive thirst, peeing and hunger. I put the thirst down to the warmth of the Floridian sun and the excessive peeing down to the amount of water I was drinking. I was feeling listless, dizzy and a bit spacey. But Florida was about to deliver a dramatic new symptom that would change everything in a heartbeat.

It was a sunny afternoon during spring break, the time when the young and the beautiful come out to party. The roads were shimmering in the heat, and I had an overwhelming urge for a doughnut. I've been travelling in southern Florida for several decades so I have some guilty pit stops—first amongst them is a large doughnut bakery in suburban Fort Lauderdale. Set back from the busy road, it's a low-rise drive-through shop with a huge sign that lights up when the doughnuts are fresh. I was 40 miles (60 kilometres) away but had nothing else to do, so I headed to Fort Lauderdale for a sugar fix.

The store was open and the light was blinking, promising freshly baked trays of doughnuts. I bought a dozen and immediately stuffed five into my face. I headed to my favourite resort, where beautiful people with bronzed bodies sat round a sparkling pool sipping martinis in the late afternoon sun. I was fat, pasty and white but I didn't care. I ordered up a jug of margarita laced with commercial cocktail mix, tequila, orange liquor and sugar and settled in for the evening. Two hours later the doughnut box sat almost empty on the bedside table and the jug of margarita had been drained.

I woke early the next morning and looked around. The world was out of focus. I staggered blurrily into the bathroom and poked at my eyes, peering into the mirror. I could sort of see some things close up, but anything more than a few inches away was just a glassy blur. I blinked and looked around the room. It was as though I'd put someone else's bottle-thick glasses on. I wandered around the room rubbing my eyes, bumping into the side of the bed and listening to the wind getting louder outside. A tropical storm was brewing. And I couldn't really see.

At the time I knew next to nothing about diabetes—in particular about how it can affect vision. There are numerous diabetic complications that can affect the eye: compromised blood vessels, retinal damage and, as in my case, temporary changes to the shape of the lens of the eye itself. I had suffered an acute shift in the refractive properties of the eye caused by a sudden spike in blood glucose that leads to blurred vision. The world around me was horribly out of focus, I was 5,000 miles from home, I couldn't really see anything, I had forgotten to renew my travel insurance and a tropical thunderstorm was raging outside.

I needed breakfast, so I reached for the last doughnut and stuffed it in my mouth. I decided to pack my gear, get into the car and drive back to the Miami airport. In my defence I was a little disorientated. The rain was torrential, making my already compromised vision even worse, and I could see almost nothing clearly. I was dizzy and a bit hysterical. I took the entire journey at 20 mph (30 kph), weaving dangerously across four-lane highways in the torrential rain. I checked into the first flight home and slept all the way back to London.

I went straight from the airport to my optician, Mohammed. He told me to go to hospital. By the end of the day I had been diagnosed with type 2 diabetes. I had a bag full of pills and a new set of temporary contact lenses that would allow me to see the world again until my eyes returned to normal.

Mohammed and I became good friends. I would go to see him every Saturday. He would take his measurements and I'd be dispatched with a new set of disposable contact lenses. After several months, my eyes stabilised and Mohammed wrote me up as an interesting case study. I owe him and the rest of the staff a huge debt of gratitude.

Other medical professionals were rather less solicitous. "You are quite fat!" my good-natured and endlessly patient diabetes nurse exclaimed one day with a mischievous smile as the tape was stretched around my midriff. "At least you are not yet obese!" was a phrase that rang in my head for many months after one particularly brutal appointment. Despite my resentment at the time, I knew she was right. Inside I was angry with everyone—with my doctors for not being able to make my diabetes go away, with supermarkets for selling me sugar-loaded junk, but mostly with myself for this self-inflicted condition.

I've often wondered if a forthright approach to medical advice is a technique to nudge patients into changing their lives, but in fact, I think it's just over-work. It must be very dispiriting to be a healthcare professional, given how many people are now presenting with type 2 diabetes. And much of what we're told as patients is true: we should stop smoking and drinking so much, we should exercise more, we should be more sensible with our diets and we should lose weight. But the relationship that many diabetes patients have with their healthcare providers can be difficult. For some it's very passive—a series of half-hearted instructions delivered without any real insight and meekly accepted by dispirited and demoralised patients. For others it's more problematic. Many of the people I've met with type 2 diabetes have experienced frustration and anxiety over the quality of the care they receive, and in some cases it boils over into activism.

There are thousands of diabetic rebels online who reject conventional treatment. Frustrated by orthodox medicine they evangelise online for a variety of natural remedies and alternative treatments or use diet alone to treat their disease. Some feel as though they are little more than passive cogs in a big-pharma machine, and there are dozens of groups on Facebook and elsewhere full of people determined to rid themselves of type 2 diabetes in their own way. Some of these online groups have tens of thousands of members, many of whom are very vocal with their advice. I lurk online but rarely participate in their furious debates.

There is a great deal of talk about ways of eating (WOE) and the pharmacological benefits of different food groups and diets. There are strong and conflicting opinions about medications, and people are regularly thrown out of some groups for saying the wrong thing or promoting alternative views to the ones championed by the group moderators. People promote remedies using dried medlar leaves or apple cider vinegar or a teaspoon of dried cinnamon or tea made from bitter melon. I've seen newcomers foolishly encouraged to double their meds or come off their pills altogether, and there are even alternative groups set up by people who have been banished from the original forums.

To be fair there is also some quiet wisdom and a great generosity of spirit on display, and I have considerable respect for people who have charted their own course to rid themselves of this disease. But ignore the folk remedies and medical suggestions from strangers on the discussion boards and go talk to your doctor in person.

I was just one of many millions of people in the system. According to Diabetes UK, since 1996 the number of people in the UK diagnosed with diabetes has more than doubled, from 1.4 million to almost 3 million. There are 700 new diagnoses a day in the UK alone and an estimated one in four people already with diabetes are actually unaware of their condition. By 2025 it's projected that more than five million people in the UK will be living with diabetes[18], and a further 11.9 million will be at an increased risk of developing it. It's a public health catastrophe on a vast scale.

It's worse for men. Almost 10 percent of men in the UK have diabetes compared with 7.6 percent of women.[19] A report[20] from November 2017 shows that men are 26 percent more likely than women to develop type 2 diabetes. Men are more likely to be overweight and to have a lower personal-fast threshold than women. Men are also less likely to admit they're overweight or participate in any kind of weight-management programme.

The cost of type 2 diabetes drugs in the UK is estimated at £700 million a year. The total cost of additional medications related to type 2 diabetes is £1.8 billion. The outpatient costs of type 2-related treatment are estimated at £1.15 billion, and the in-patient costs associated with diabetic complications are estimated at a staggering £8 billion. Ten percent of all NHS primary care prescribing in the UK is now for diabetes, and by 2035 it is predicted that it could cost the NHS £17 billion a year. That's about the same amount of money that the Brexiteers told us could be recycled back into the NHS if we left the EU.

The picture is even worse elsewhere in the world. The US has the

---

18 Diabetic Prevalence Model PHE (https://www.gov.uk/government/news/38-million-people-in-england-now-have-diabetes)

19 Diabetic Prevalence Model PHE (https://www.gov.uk/government/news/38-million-people-in-england-now-have-diabetes)

20 https://www.menshealthforum.org.uk/one-ten-male-diabetes-crisis

highest prevalence of diabetes amongst all developed countries in the world. The statistics are eye-watering. Almost 11 percent of people between the ages of 20 and 79 in the US have diabetes—that's more than 30 million adults. A further 84 million people—almost a third of the entire population— are estimated to have pre-diabetes, and of those only 11.5 percent actually know they have it. One and a half million new cases are diagnosed in the US each year[21]. Such is the scale of the epidemic that the US has nearly two-thirds of the total number of cases of all of the other 37 developed nations of the world combined. And there are 50 other countries where the incidence of diabetes is more than 10 percent of the total adult population, including Bahrain, Kuwait, Singapore, Malaysia, Saudi Arabia, Mexico, Turkey and Egypt.

These days I cannot pass a doughnut stall without a wry smile, but I walk right past. I make no direct connection between eating a dozen doughnuts in one sitting and my diagnosis. My diabetes crept up on me because of decades of poor eating habits and self-indulgent lifestyle choices.

Doughnuts are now dead to me. But as much as I miss them, the doughnut industry hasn't missed me very much. Doughnut shops have blossomed on high streets and in shopping malls worldwide. National Doughnut Day is celebrated in North America on the first Friday of June each year, and at least one major chain was due to open over 350 new stores in the US alone in 2018. The global doughnut market was worth $40 billion in 2016 and is projected to reach $55 billion by 2024.

That's great news for the shareholders of the major doughnut manufacturers; I'm rather less sure how good it is for the rest of us.

---

21 https://www.cdc.gov/media/releases/2017/p0718-diabetes-report.html

THE DIAGNOSIS

One day you think you're perfectly healthy and the next you have a chronic "lifelong" medical condition. Frankly, it's a shock.

I've come across people who have responded very badly to a diabetic or pre-diabetic diagnosis, with anger, shame, denial, indignation and depression. For me it was confusion. Diabetes was something other people got—old people, or people who were born with it, or people who had to inject themselves every day. Not me. Of all the advice I got when I was first diagnosed, none of it focused on my psychological response to this chronic illness, despite the clear incidence of mental-health needs amongst newly diagnosed patients.

There's a really important reason why our psychological response is important. Much of what we're told as newly diagnosed patients is about clinical treatment, medications and advice about the lifestyle changes we must make. But time is short in a diabetes clinic, and much of the advice comes in the form of poorly printed materials and by-the-book conversations about being healthy and getting more exercise. No one ever raised the prospect of being able to overcome the diagnosis; the advice I got was all about the pills and check-ups with a little lifestyle advice thrown in.

The challenges of managing this disease have given birth to a condition recognised as "diabetes-related distress," a raft of psychological symptoms, including depression, frustration around taking medications, skipping consultations and check-ups and a profound feeling of being overwhelmed or defeated by the diagnosis. I recognised many of these issues: I hated taking the pills, I definitely wanted more from my medical advisors and I was inconsistent about keeping appointments.

My advice to any newly diagnosed patient would be to talk to your doctor about how to manage the disease beyond the pills and the annual tests. Ask what you can do to stay on top of the diagnosis and what, if anything, you can do to overcome it? Check yourself if you have the urge to skip an appointment. Be honest with yourself about the other factors in your life that might have a bearing on your diagnosis and talk to other people who have the same condition. And if you can, find others who have conquered the disease and talk to them about how they did it.

I regret wasting several years belligerently doing what I was told, taking the pills and trying to change my diet without any clear focus. I was told I would be on the pills for life and that daily injections were probably coming, so what was the point of challenging it? As long as it didn't get any worse, the medical profession was telling me that I just had to improve my lifestyle and take the meds. My blood tests did improve a little in the early years but never to such a point that I could be classified as diabetes-free. And I did lose a little weight by cutting out some indulgences over the years, probably about six to eight kilos. But I was hardly scratching the surface of this life-changing condition. Like many others, I was simply accepting it as my destiny.

THE NUMBERS

Test results become a way of life when you are first diagnosed. There are lots of numbers attached to diabetes. As well as fasting blood glucose levels and HbA1c tests, there are cholesterol tests, blood pressure tests, oral glucose tolerance tests, urine tests, eye tests and foot exams. But, for me, there were only two important things to focus on: HbA1c and fasting blood glucose.

HbA1c

Normal:	*below 5.7% (39mmol/mol)*
Pre-diabetes:	*5.7%–6.4% (39mmol/mol–46.4mmol/mol)*
Diabetes:	*6.5% (48mmol/mol) or higher*

An HbA1c test (known as A1C in the US) measures your recent average blood glucose levels. Measuring the glucose attached to part of the red blood cells gives a good indication of the effectiveness of blood sugar control during the preceding two to three months. The advantage of this test is that you don't have to fast before taking it. Two numbers can come with an HbA1C test—a percentage score or an actual number. Older DCCT-aligned (percentages) and newer IFCC-standardised (mmol/mol) concentrations can be compared in the table from www.wales.nhs – see reference below[22]. Conversions are grouped according to each percentage point on the current DCCT-aligned measurement scale, and IFCC-standardised values are rounded to the nearest whole number. An HbA1c score above 6.5 percent (48mmol/mol) is a diabetic score. I scored a strikingly unhealthy 14.9 percent (139.3mmol/mol).

Fasting blood glucose

Normal:	*below 5.5mmol/L (100mg/dL)*
Pre-diabetes:	*5.5mmol/L–6.9mmol/L (100g/dL–125mg/dL)*
Diabetes:	*7mmol/L or higher (126mg/dL)*

A fasting blood glucose test measures blood glucose after fasting

---

22 http://www.wales.nhs.uk/sitesplus/documents/866/HbA1c%20converter.pdf

for at least eight hours. It's used to test the effectiveness of different medications or dietary changes for people already diagnosed as diabetic or at risk of developing the disease. There are two units often used to describe this score. In Europe it's more common to use mmol/L, and in the United States, people tend to use a mg/dL scale. A score of 7mmol/L (126mg/dL) or higher on two separate occasions indicates diabetes. I was a whopping 23mmol/L (414mg/dL).

Intermediate scores put people in a pre-diabetic range that indicates a risk of developing full-blown type 2 diabetes in the future. Doctors sometimes refer to pre-diabetes as impaired glucose tolerance (IGT) or impaired fasting glucose (IFG), depending on which test is used. It points to the fact that a patient's diet, exercise and lifestyle need some close attention. But the term pre-diabetes is not without controversy. Supporters of the term argue that it allows for the efficient classification of high-risk patients so there can be some early intervention to prevent the onset of full-blown diabetes. Others complain about both the definition and impact of a pre-diabetic score and even invoke the hidden hand of big pharma, keen to drive sales and institutionalising a problem that doesn't need pharmaceutical intervention.

Frankly I don't care about such politics, and I don't understand the science well enough to have a view. I simply don't want to be diabetic or even pre-diabetic. I want to be on the right side of an absolute set of numbers. And I really don't want to take the pills.

As I sat with my doctor reviewing my first test results in March 2012, I saw the concern on her face. I was only half-listening to the numbers. Phrases like "off the scale" and "sky high" danced across my consciousness. It was all a bit of a blur. She mused on how long I had actually had diabetes without knowing and wondered how much higher my results would have been if I'd been tested the morning I woke up in Florida. Words like "diabetic coma" floated past me as she reflected on the severity of my scores.

My condition had incubated during years of poor lifestyle choices, overindulgence and irresponsible idleness. It took me five years to find the resolve to do something about it, but since I'd discovered the Newcastle study, I sat down to work out how I could get rid of the internal fat that I assumed was inhibiting my internal organ function.

It was a decision that was to change my life.

THE PLAN

In order to work for me, my plan needed to be simple and straightforward. I settled on five rules that would come to dominate my approach to dealing with the diagnosis. Each has worthwhile benefits in itself, but together they produced some startling results. For this to have a chance of working my plan was to:

1. Reduce daily carbohydrate loads

2. Eliminate all refined sugars and reduce other sugars as much as possible

3. Reduce daily calorie intake for a limited period

4. Drink more water

5. And undertake some light exercise.

These five key issues—carbs, calories, sugars, water consumption and exercise—are all covered later in this section, together with some other topics. As simple as they sound, experience taught me that in practice they can be a huge challenge, and it takes single-minded determination and a degree of self-discipline to stick to them.

I acknowledge that these five core rules won't be popular with everyone. There are those who believe that increasing water intake is modish mumbo jumbo and that achieving a minimum number of steps each day is an Internet myth with no scientific evidence to back it up. Other people don't advise restricting calories for any length of time and many keep a much wider range of sugars in their diet than I chose to keep. But these five simple rules worked for me. Weaning myself off sugar was important to overcome my addiction to short-term sugar fixes, and undertaking some light exercise and drinking more water helped in the many ways listed later in this chapter. Temporary calorie reduction was also important, not least because it brought some discipline to my out-of-control greed. Of course I don't know if my outcome would have changed had I chosen only to stick to one or two of these rules, but I'm not sure that any of them in isolation would have delivered the transformation I was after.

What l landed on was a modified version of the classic Banting diet, a low-carbohydrate, high-fat regime named after William Banting, a 19th century undertaker who dropped a significant amount of his body weight. Mr Banting was so delighted with his physical transformation that he wrote a pamphlet, *Letter on Corpulance, Addressed to the Public,* which did modestly well in several editions. It's freely available online,[23] and it's a marvellous, if rather idiosyncratic, read. It went on to inspire a whole host of subsequent dietary experts, including the Real Meal Revolution championed by Professor Tim Noakes and supposedly the now-ubiquitous Atkins diet.

A low-carb regime prompts your body into switching from burning carbs for energy to burning fat to promote weight loss. The theory of a very low-carb Banting diet is that if people eat the right types of fats and minimal carbs (typically avoiding anything with a carb content of more than 5g per 100g and cutting out most sugar) then they can eat reasonable portion sizes. My modified low-carb diet was rather more generous with carb content. I set myself a limit of foods that were lower than 10g per 100g serving, but I traded off the higher carb

---

23 https://archive.or g/details/letteroncorpulen00bant

limit by restricting my portion sizes and by temporarily cutting my calories below the limits of the classic Banting diet. Calorie reduction is a contested subject for reasons that become clear later (*see page 49*).

Banting's original diet also allowed for prodigious quantities of alcohol. He allowed for two or three glasses of good claret, sherry, or Madeira at lunchtime (although to give him credit, champagne, port and beer were forbidden), a "glass or two" of claret at supper and a tumbler of grog (gin, whisky, or brandy) or another "glass or two" of claret or sherry before going to bed. My version allows for none of these things.

There are many variations of a low-carb diet, and I'm the first to admit that what I'm proposing here is very far from original. There are many versions of what I did, and some of them may be better for you; I simply changed some essential details to make it a bit more straightforward and achievable for me. Some plans measure net carbs (where you subtract the fibre from the carb load) and others have you pace yourself through the day using carefully measured carb loads. For example, the Bernstein 6/12/12 plan for the treatment of type 1 diabetes, developed by endocrinologist and type 1 diabetic Richard K. Bernstein and first published in 1997, limits patients to 6g of carbs for breakfast and 12g each for lunch and dinner.

There is also a difference between a low-carb diet and a keto diet. If you normally eat 300g of carbohydrates a day and shift to 80g or 100g a day, you're following a lower-carbohydrate diet. There are all sorts of variations of low-carb regimes: the ubiquitous Paleo diet, the Atkins method, the South Beach diet, the low-carb Mediterranean diet and many others.

A keto diet is a significantly tougher version of a low-carb diet in which people aim to achieve a state of nutritional ketosis by consuming less than 30g of carbs a day (some would say even less) and replacing the missing carbs with higher natural fats. Achieving nutritional ketosis, however, is fraught with difficulties; it's not as simple as "what goes in comes off." Different people have different thresholds for achieving a state of ketosis. Maintaining a ketogenic diet in the long term is a considerable undertaking and can provoke some challenging side effects, including flu-like symptoms, headaches, irritability, lethargy, difficulties in concentration and leg cramps, unless you know exactly what you're doing. There were certainly times when I achieved ketosis on this regime, but I was insufficiently disciplined to be on a ruthlessly ketogenic diet for the whole five months.

The plan I used has five sections. The first is week zero, the "baseline" week, followed by four periods of changing food habits, each lasting for four weeks—sixteen weeks in total. Then there was a "landing" period, where I returned to a "normal" diet with some enduring long-term changes that I'd become acclimatised to over the months.

PREPARATION: WEEK ZERO

Week zero is all about preparation. There is no diet this week, as it's all about understanding and preparing for the big changes ahead. The knowledge I gleaned in this week fuelled everything else that was to come, and it became the measure against which I set all my targets for the next few months. This is also the week where you must get some professional medical advice from your doctor or a qualified nutritionist or dietitian.

Simple things, like setting a final-weight target, deciding my daily calorie and carb limits and setting a target daily step count, were all decided in week zero. Here is the list of the 10 key things that needed to happen that week:

1. Keeping a thorough daily food diary recording everything I ate—no cheating and no kidding myself. This daily food diary revealed the hideous truth of my eye-watering daily calorie, sugar and carbohydrate loads.

2. Recording all my daily physical activity. I used the health app preloaded on my iPhone to automatically record my daily steps and other activity. The baseline week demonstrated just how inactive I was. Activity trackers are ubiquitous on all smartphones, and some people wear portable fitness trackers.

3. Weighing in. Dispiriting, right? I chose to weigh myself daily, which is not popular with many professionals for reasons that are discussed later (*see page 41*). But I got used to it, and at the end of this week I set my final target weight range.

4. Getting an up-to-date set of blood results from my medical advisor. If you are going to attempt something similar, it is critical that you talk to your medical provider about the wisdom of undertaking this regime given your own circumstances, including a discussion about the impact of a low-carb diet on the medications you take.

5. Setting a progressive temporary calorie deficit (*see page 49*), and a daily carbohydrate target (*see page 44*) linked to an ultimate weight goal, both decided in close collaboration with your medical advisor.

6. Preparing to change portion sizes.

7. Banishing all sugars, pastas, potatoes, flour, rice, bread, crisps, sweets, snacks, biscuits, crackers, cartons of fruit juice and fruit concentrates from the cupboard and buying the ingredients for the first week's meals.

8. Getting used to the fact that from the next week forward, there wasn't to be any alcohol. It would come back later, but for now it was out.

9. Planning how to achieve an activity target of at least 10,000 steps a day.

10. Increasing my water intake to at least 2½ litres/4½ pints per day.

Cooking for, or regularly eating with, other people can add significant pressures to this plan. There are two options to this: either they can join you in the journey, or you'll start to eat quite different things. It is very possible to do this diet with your family by modifying your own plate at mealtimes. You simply remove the things that aren't allowed on your regime. But to achieve success on this regime, the family diet may need to change, or, at least for part of the time, you may end up preparing different things to eat for yourself.

Talk it through with the people you live with. Be very clear—are you going to do this together? Or are you going to modify your own diet and eat different stuff? Make the decision with them, and ask them for their help. They will want you to succeed. They will want you to be well, but make it clear that their 100 percent support will be absolutely crucial to your success.

A FOOD DIARY

To shortcut the laborious process of measuring food and hand writing a food diary, I managed this entire process on a smartphone. I used Virtuagym's Calorie, Carb and Fat Counter, an awesomely clever free app. It is one of many such free applications, and it takes the hard work out of keeping a manual food diary. During the setup, it asks if you wish to link it to the Health app on an iPhone. Use it to record everything that you eat. If you'd prefer to do it the old-fashioned way, you can find helpful resources and links to help with this at conquertype2diabetes.com.

Ruthless honesty is needed when recording a food diary. According to the UK's Office for National Statistics, a third of adults underestimate how much they eat[24]. A study of 4,000 people over a four-day period revealed that some men routinely eat 3,000 calories or more a day when they claim to be eating only 2,000 calories. Some

---

24 https://datasciencecampus.ons.gov.uk/2017/11/08/how-much-is-the-uk-eating/

women say they eat 1,500 calories a day, when the truth is that they eat closer to 2,500 calories. That's 50 percent more than the recommended daily allowance for most people.

The results of keeping a daily food diary and activity diary in week zero may be a little shocking—they were for me. I was indolent (doing less than 3,000 steps a day), overweight (117 kilos) and eating way too much (between 3,000 and 4,000 calories and often more than 400g of carbs each day). At least half of my diet was based on carbs, and I was eating monumental amounts of refined sugar. All of this had to change.

WEIGHT TARGET

Setting an ultimate weight target can be something like a life sentence, so settling on an ideal result is an important decision. It can become a measure by which people define themselves and can cause considerable self-esteem issues if it's so unrealistic that it's always out of reach.

Instead of settling on an absolute number, I ended up choosing a final target range. Apparently my "ideal" body weight is 12 st 9 lb/82.5kg and the "healthy" range for a man of my age and height is between 10 st 5 lb/66.8kg and 14 st 2 lb/90.6kg. You can calculate your own range by using the NHS BMI Healthy Weight Calculator[25] online or by checking out conquertype2diabetes.com.

An absolute "ideal" weight score can be very disheartening. There's no one I know who hasn't looked at the charts and been anything other than indignant when they discovered their "ideal" weight. I've never been my ideal weight, and I'm sure I never will be. The lowest I ever actually got was 13 st 4 lb/85.2kg, but it's never really been about an "ideal" body weight for me. It's about getting rid of enough fat to restore my natural pancreatic and liver function, and everyone's personal fat thresholds are different.

---

25 https://www.nhs.uk/Tools/Pages/Healthyweightcalculator.aspx

I knew that when I finally returned to normal eating, my weight would likely fluctuate, so I cut myself some slack. When I started the process, I was just over 18 st 4 lb/117kg. I decided that I'd settle for between 13 st 3 lb and 13 st 8 lb/85 and 88kg, even if that meant I wasn't going to be "ideal" according to the textbooks.

As I write these words, I'm 13 st 8 lb/88kg, which makes me close to being borderline overweight. But it's easy to forget that this process isn't about being "overweight" or "normal"—this is about *not being diabetic*. I may be close to being overweight, but I'm not diabetic, so I'll live with being that close to the line.

The scales are your friends, mostly. People have different views about weighing themselves regularly. Many people will tell you (for very good reasons) not to do it every day. And there are others, like me, who simply can't stop weighing themselves daily. Notwithstanding the advice from many trainers and self-help books, I made the decision to record my weight at the same time every day, and it's a habit that lasts to this day.

I took some inspiration from being able to summon up weekly and monthly weight charts and watch the progress. It worked as an incentive for me, and it gave me a sense of purpose to see what was happening. I weighed myself as soon as I got up, before breakfast and without clothes, every morning and popped the result into the app on my phone. Doing it weekly is just fine for most people.

It can also be quite gratifying at the start of the process. For the first six to eight weeks, if you respond as I did, chances are that you may see some encouraging early progress. There is, however, a law of diminishing returns. The weight-loss curve is steep at the start and much, much shallower towards the end of the programme. Losing the first kilo is much more straightforward than losing the last. However, a daily weigh-in habit comes with a big health warning about water retention.

WATER

There were simple, practical reasons why it was important for me to drink more water on this low-carb approach: it helped to make me feel full and counteracted the grumblings of an empty stomach; it helped avoid constipation and counteracted the production of dark, burning urine, which can come with dieting, and ketosis in particular; and I also found that it helped with digestion. Before starting this diet, my daily fluids came from strong espresso coffee, high-sugar fruit juices and alcohol. Now, water has become an important refreshing and healthy alternative.

Rather than carrying around a water bottle, I made regular appointments with water every single day. I drank a large glass first thing in the morning, after the weigh-in but before eating breakfast. The second glass of water came as soon as I arrived in the office, and I had another immediately before lunch. And I drink chilled, sparkling water with my main evening meal. Consuming 2.5 litres/4½ pints of water per day sounded a lot when I first started, but now it's a simple, healthy habit. Plan the times when you will drink water, and stick to it ruthlessly.

Water retention can play havoc with a daily weigh-in. It will skew daily weight results to a far greater degree than any weight loss associated with fat reduction in the short term. It's entirely possible to be losing weight through fat loss while it seems that you're putting on weight, simply because of the way the body retains water. If you're planning to weigh yourself every day, bear in mind that week-to-week and month-to-month changes are much more important than the daily changes or the plateaus, which can be very dispiriting and are often attributable to water retention rather than any underlying weight loss from fat reduction.

CARBOHYDRATES

This regime was based first and foremost on a dramatic reduction in daily carbohydrate load and refined sugars. Temporarily reducing calorie intake was only a short-lived process for me, and if you respond in the same way I did, the most important parts of this programme (reducing the daily carb load, cutting back on sugar, increasing water intake and modestly raising activity levels) are likely to stay with you much longer than any temporary reduction in calories.

Remember that some diabetes medications (including insulin) need very careful monitoring on a low-carb diet. Some sulfonylureas (minidiab, euglucon, daonil, and glibenclamide) can provoke very low blood sugars on a low-carb diet. And drugs known as SLGT2 inhibitors can trigger very unwelcome side effects, including ketoacidosis, on a low-carb regime. A low-carb diet can also provoke unwelcome side effects for people on blood pressure medication and for women who are breastfeeding. Do not start a low-carb diet without consulting your physician. Tell your doctor what you're planning and ask explicitly if you should remain on the same medication regime.

Restricting carbohydrates is a hotly contested subject in both the UK and the United States. The online message groups are full of stories of people being told to maintain a low-fat, high-carb diet by their medical advisors, but neither the National Health Service in the UK nor the American Diabetes Association vigorously endorses a dramatic reduction in carb intake for people who want to reverse their diagnosis. For me, it is the only way to go. Carbohydrates need to be dramatically and ruthlessly reduced for this regime to have any chance of working.

My relationship with carbohydrates might be unusual in that I may be more carb-intolerant than others. I have friends who can hoover their way through piles of croissants, potatoes, pizza, rice and pasta and stay as thin as a rake. If I stuff myself with carbs, I see an almost immediate effect. My daily weigh-in goes haywire, and I feel fat, bloated, listless and sluggish the next day. But if I banish carbs from my diet, many of those things simply evaporate.

The NHS warns us that reducing carbs makes fibre consumption more challenging, fibre being important for a healthy digestive system. It warns that it can put people at an increased risk of essential nutritional deficiencies, and we're told that there is a risk from the increased saturated fats of raising cholesterol levels and contributing to the risk of heart disease. And ketosis (which sometimes comes with very low-carb diets) can lead to headaches, nausea, irritability, dehydration and dizziness[26].

It all sounds terrifying, doesn't it? It's really not. To be clear, while I'm losing weight, I want my body to lose the excess fat I'm carrying. I can replace the nutrients I need from other, much healthier sources. The process of dropping weight can have some irksome side effects, but you can compensate for them by focusing on a diet of healthy foods, including lots of fresh green vegetables, fruits and berries, natural dairy products, meat and seafood.

Of course some people have reported a range of side effects, including the well-known bad-breath syndrome that can come with ketosis, constipation, leg cramps, low energy levels, unusually cold feet and hands and insomnia. I've had some of these, but they weren't so overpowering that they changed my life, and all of them disappeared after a while. If you are concerned about any of these side effects, check with your doctor.

There are some doctors who will advise you to ease gradually into a low-carb diet to ameliorate some of the side effects, but my experience was that they weren't sufficiently strong or worrying to do this. Cutting out carbs in itself is unlikely to lead to any significant vitamin deficiency, assuming that you consume a wide range of

26 https://www.nhs.uk/Livewell/loseweight/Pages/the-truth-about-carbs.aspx

alternative healthy foods. I added a daily sugar-free multivitamin to my diet, but a wide range of fresh vegetables, the right fruits, natural dairy products, meat, fish and other seafood provided me with everything I needed to both stay healthy and lose weight.

Not all carbs are created equal; some carbs are unavoidable and are good for you, others not so much. For the purposes of this regime, however, all processed carbs and other starchy foods and all flour products, such as bread, crackers, pastries, biscuits, cakes, pasta, rice (including wholegrain rice), potatoes and all refined sugars, simply need to go. Some purists choose to record their net carb intake rather than their total carb intake. Net carbs are simply the grams of total carbohydrates in a portion of food, minus its grams of fibre. Because fibre is a carbohydrate that your body can't digest, it doesn't raise your blood sugar levels to the same degree or trigger an insulin response. I didn't do such convoluted calculations—life is just too short.

I missed many of the psychological joys that come with carbohydrates. I craved the mouthfeel that comes with a high-carb diet—crispy toast, flaky pastry, fresh crusty bread, fluffy roasted potatoes, velvety rice and creamy pasta are all joyous high notes in the music of food. But for now, get used to it—they're out. They'll be back in modest quantities later, but right now you have a bigger challenge than fixing the craving for a freshly baked baguette. You're here to get rid of type 2 diabetes, right?

My simple rule of thumb was that any product that had a score of more than 10g of carbs per 100g on the label was ejected from the shopping basket. I had set myself a relatively low daily carb target on this programme. And since it's very, very tricky to skip carbs altogether, I settled on a total carb limit of between 40g and 60g a day, which is close to a ketogenic threshold, but you can choose any daily carb target you and your nutritionist decide. In general, for this plan to be effective, it needs to be at the lower end of the range; anything more than 80g of carbs a day may not deliver the results you want.

And as I did my weekly shop, I focused my vegetable selection on vegetables that grow above the ground rather than below ground. This might seem like a bit of a random rule, but I found it incredibly useful as I stared blankly at the supermarket shelves wondering what I could actually eat. Spinach, kale, green beans, courgette (zucchini), cabbage, asparagus, cucumber, okra, avocado, broccoli, spinach and cauliflower are all great vegetables for a low-carb diet. Some above-the-ground vegetables, like corn and peas, were (irritatingly) too high in carbs for me on this diet. And many root vegetables like potatoes, parsnips, yams, beetroot and sweet potatoes were also off the list because of their high-starch, high-carb content. At the start of this regime, I assumed that I might be eating lots of beans and pulses, but I banished red beans, lentils and quinoa from my shopping list because of their carb counts. Edamame beans were the one delicious exception to this.

I studied the lists of "bad" and "good" vegetables carefully on the various websites dedicated to low-carb recipes and took exception to the fact that for some people, carrots and onions appeared on the wrong side of the line simply because they were root vegetables. I decided this was ridiculous, and I kept them in. Radishes, which are also root vegetables, were great for my version of this diet. And of course there are other exceptions to the below-ground rule. Celeriac (also known as turnip-rooted celery, celery root or knob celery), for example, is a root vegetable that I concluded was fine for my version of this low-carb diet, and I used it as a mash substitute on many occasions.

Nuts were tricky. Some nuts are great, others not so much. Chestnuts were out for their carb-busting content, but I didn't mind as they're not my favourite. So were cashews, sadly, which I minded much more. The best news was that macadamia nuts, peanuts, pistachios, walnuts and pecans were all fine for carbs but again, only in small quantities, as a small handful of nuts (15g to 18g/0.5 oz) is very roughly 100 calories.

NATURAL FATS

We're told that fat, especially saturated fat, is bad for you and that fat is the primary cause of obesity and weight gain. That's not my experience. A diet high in carbs, particularly processed carbohydrates and refined sugars, led me into obesity and almost certainly contributed to the onset of my diabetes. But in general, this diet doesn't cut out the natural fats, which we've been told are bad for us for so many years. Indeed, there are real advantages to eating natural, full-fat foods on a low-carbohydrate diet and like many others, the approach I took was actually to selectively increase my natural fat intake as my daily carb load went down.

Instead of choosing low-fat products, I started reading the labels on packaged foods. I'd committed to reducing carbs, and many low-fat varieties of foods actually have more carbs in them than the full-fat versions. Low-fat cream cheese, for example, has 15 percent carbs, whereas regular cream cheese has 4 percent carbs. In fact, cheese was one of the greatest revelations on this regime. Many cheeses, including soft and medium-soft goat's cheeses, have next to no carbs in them at all, and feta, brie, Cheddar, Gruyère, mozzarella and Parmesan cheeses are all fine for a low-carb regime.

A 6-ounce serving of whole-milk Greek yoghurt has 7 percent carbs, whereas the same size portion of non-fat or skimmed milk yoghurt can have 13 percent carbs—more if it's laced with fruit flavours. And since I was banishing the carbs, I generally went for the natural full-fat versions.

The medical profession doesn't universally welcome this approach, and I watched a discussion group get extremely animated about the benefits and disadvantages of a low-carb/high-fat approach to eating. The abusive term "butter-chuggers" is online shorthand for people who champion this approach. Regular cholesterol checks become very important if you're going to diet in this way. Tests of your total cholesterol and triglyceride levels are likely to become part of the battery of tests your doctor will ask for after your diagnosis and as you undertake any significant change in diet. Both my total cholesterol and triglyceride scores were at unhealthy levels when I was first diagnosed in 2012.

Friends told me that even if I managed to bring my blood glucose to normal non-diabetic levels, a diet high in natural fats put me in danger of swapping diabetes for the perils of elevated cholesterol and potential heart disease. But I stubbornly stuck to the plan, relying on natural fats as a source of fuel to replace the carbs I had banished. In late summer 2017, after the weight loss was over, I went through a battery of tests to check my cholesterol and triglycerides.

My total cholesterol score came in at 2.58mmol/L[27] (down from 6.2mmol/L when I was first diagnosed) and my triglycerides had plummeted to 1.22mmol/L (from a high of 9.4mmol/L upon diagnosis). Blood pressure scores showed a similar trajectory: In 2011, my blood pressure was 146/96, and by August 2017 it was 121/73.

CALORIES

The primary reason I added a short-term calorie reduction to this programme was that my eating habits had become quite compulsive. If I liked something, I would binge on vast quantities of it. I might

---

27 A normal total cholesterol level should be below 5mmol/L and a healthy fasting triglyceride score should be below 1.7mmol/L. In the UK all cholesterol levels are measured in millimoles per litre (mmol/L), but in some countries they are measured in milligrams per decilitre (mg/dL). Heart UK, the UK's cholesterol charity, provides a useful formula for converting between scores used in the UK and those used in other countries, including the USA at https://heartuk.org.uk/files/uploads/documents/huk_fs_mfsP_cholestrigly_leverls-conversion.pdf

be eating a relatively low-carb food, but I would eat a lot of it. For example, salted peanuts have 6g of carbs per 100g serving, which means they had a place on my diet. But the temptation to eat a lot of them was overwhelming; the same 100g of peanuts has 615 calories, and I would think nothing of eating an entire large bag in one evening—that's well over 1,000 calories. Pork scratchings (pork rinds or cracklings) are similar: zero carbs, so great, but high in calories, 550 calories per 100g. In addition to being high in calories, they're loaded with salt. Eat them if you really must, but only in very limited quantities.

A normal man of my height and with my activity levels typically needs around 2,500 calories a day to function; women need around 2,000 calories a day. In week zero of my programme, I discovered I was eating on average between 3,000 and 4,000 calories a day. To put this in perspective, one large fresh bread from my local Indian takeaway restaurant contains 550 calories. It's pretty easy to eat your entire calorie load in one fast-food meal or by snacking, even on low-carb foods.

A glazed doughnut contains 200 calories. A 350mL/12 fl oz margarita on the rocks has 680 calories in it, mostly thanks to the sugar–syrup mix and the sweet orange liquor. Looking back, I suspect that my Florida doughnut and margarita fest contained at least 4,000 calories. And that didn't include an IHOP cheeseburger omelette I'd eaten earlier the same day. It was an awesome combination of hamburger, hash browns, tomatoes, onions, cheese, ketchup, mustard and pickles that was served with three buttermilk pancakes and syrup on the side, which apparently comes in at a whopping 1,990 calories.

For many people, losing weight simply means calorie counting; however, for me calorie restriction was combined with a low-carb approach not least because it helped contain my own unattractive, long-standing predisposition to greed. Exercise was also important, but infuriatingly, exercise uses only a small proportion of the daily calories we consume: One hour of moderate exercise, such as brisk walking, will perhaps burn 100 to 200 calories. I did it because it made me feel better, rather than for the effect it had on weight loss.

If you choose to include a short-term calorie reduction in your programme, the extent and duration of the deficit is up to you and your health advisor. I used a simple progressive formula that was ruthless (some would say *too* ruthless) at the start and became gradually more relaxed over time. I did this over four blocks, each lasting for four weeks, and planned for a progressively less-ruthless calorie deficit in each block. Here's the formula I used:

- Weeks 1 through 4: a calorie limit of 1,650 calories a day (66 percent of my normal calorie intake)
- Weeks 5 through 8: a calorie limit of 1,900 calories a day (75 percent of my normal calorie intake)
- Weeks 9 through 12: a calorie limit of 2,100 calories a day (85 percent of my normal calorie intake)
- Weeks 13 through 16: a calorie limit of 2,250 calories a day (90 percent of my normal calorie intake)

If you choose to include a short-term calorie restriction, picking the right deficit is a very important decision. Too small, and there will not be enough impact early on to sustain your motivation. But pick too great a deficit, and it can be extremely unhealthy and even dangerous. At the risk of being repetitious, this is another moment when you must seek help from a doctor, a professional nutritionist or a personal trainer, and the calculation of what's right for you might be very different from what worked for me.

There are several freely available apps that you can use to monitor your daily calorie, fat and carb intake. The setup sequence will guide you through the options to achieve your ideal daily loads, and it will also factor in your weight-loss aspirations. Each day, you record what you've eaten, and it calculates how well you're doing against the plan and how close you are to achieving your daily targets. You can also use it to explore your daily and weekly consumption and monitor your weight progress. There are simple copy/paste functions that allow you to copy meals from one day to another.

There will be days when it all goes horribly wrong. Instead of achieving my target carb and calorie intakes, I sometimes flew way over them. If the same happens to you, don't be disheartened, but understand where you cheated and check yourself the next day. The whole process of recording food consumption takes a few minutes at the start and end of each day, but the investment of time is vital if you're going to get clear insight into your progress.

UNWELCOME SIDE EFFECTS

There is strong evidence that severely restricting calories over an extended period of time can precipitate psychological complications for some people and can even lead to eating disorders. The Minnesota Starvation Experiment, which ran from 1944 to 1945, saw a group of male volunteers undertake a three-step programme: a 12-week control phase (with a 'normal' diet of 3500kcal per day) during which observations were collected; a 24-week 'starvation' phase (1570kcal per day) during which participants lost an average of 25 percent of their pre-starvation body weight; and finally a recovery phase in which the volunteers returned to a normal nourishing diet.

The results of the study were salutary. Many of the volunteers saw decreases in their strength and stamina, body temperature, heart rate and sex drive. Hunger drove the men to become obsessed with food as they dreamed and fantasised about it. In addition, many reported periods of fatigue, irritability, depression and apathy, and in some cases, the psychological and behavioural effects lasted well into the recovery phase and long after participants had regained their original weight.

What I was doing hardly felt like starvation. I was eating healthy, nutritious food and rarely felt hungry. In hindsight, I did perhaps experience one or two of these symptoms (I was irritable sometimes, and I did dream about cream cakes more than once), but these side effects were only fleeting. I became a little more reclusive than I had been previously (although according to my close friends I'm famously antisocial anyway so it was quite hard to spot). And I did at times become preoccupied with food, but mostly this came in the form of being inexcusably smug and boring with my friends as I listed the carbohydrate values of my daily diet and irritatingly urged others to stop eating cake.

Fifty-seven years after the experiment, in 2018, researchers published a follow-up study[28] involving 19 of the original volunteers. At the time of the follow up, they were aged between 75 and 83. Many reported maintaining a higher than normal weight in the years after the experiment, and some had experienced abnormal eating habits for many months, and even years, before returning to 'normal'. The researchers concluded, however, that the volunteers' experience was not associated with lifelong physical, cognitive or emotional adverse effects, despite the significant challenges they had experienced during the experiment.

Nevertheless, this is a clear warning: seek professional medical advice as you go through this regime. Seeing body fat fall away is a gratifying physical change, but this can mask more challenging

---

28 https://www.researchgate.net/profile/Regina_Casper/
publication/324507398_A_57-YEAR_FOLLOW-UP_INVESTI-
GATION_AND_REVIEW_OF_THE_MINNESOTA_STUDY_ON_HU-
MAN_STARVATION_AND_ITS_RELEVANCE_TO_EATING_DISORDERS/
links/5ad14934aca272fdaf7797ca/A-57-YEAR-FOLLOW-UP-INVESTIGATION-AND-
REVIEW-OF-THE-MINNESOTA-STUDY-ON-HUMAN-STARVATION-AND-ITS-RELEVANCE-TO-
EATING-DISORDERS.pdf?origin=publication_list

psychological and physiological side effects that only a medical professional or a very strong social network might be able to spot, whether it be anorexia nervosa or another eating disorder.

An unhealthy preoccupation with the 'right' kind of food can in itself become a challenge for some. Fifty years after the Minnesota experiment, the term 'orthorexia' was coined to describe a condition where a restrictive diet (often an obsession with 'pure' or 'clean' food) leads to unhealthy consequences, disordered eating and, in some cases, malnutrition. Despite widespread media interest, orthorexia is not widely recognised and the medical profession has not adopted it as a formal diagnosis.

I didn't have a pathological obsession with eating 'proper' or 'pure' foods, and although I think it's unlikely that I was orthorexic, one sign of the condition made me wince in hindsight: 'Because it requires considerable willpower to adopt a diet that differs radically from the food habits of childhood and the surrounding culture,' says the originator of the term, Dr Steven Bratman, 'few accomplish the change gracefully. Most must resort to an iron self-discipline bolstered by a hefty dose of superiority over those who eat junk food.'[29] Looking back, I know that I had become single-minded in my approach to food, and it started to dominate my conversation and some parts of my life. I did start to feel unpleasantly superior to people who I saw eating fast food or loading their shopping baskets with high-carb products.

The multiple psychological benefits that come with weight loss can mask some unexpected consequences. As people lose weight, they inevitably attract comments from friends and family; constantly being told how well you're doing and how healthy you look can become addictive. Repeated positive affirmation from friends and family can fuel a deep-seated dissatisfaction with body image issues long after reasonable weight loss has been achieved.

---

29 p. 47, Yoga Journal, September/October 1997

For me, redemption came from the Kitchen Guru, who helpfully made a thoughtful intervention one late summer afternoon when she told me that enough was enough. I was being boring, she announced, and actually I was thin enough. It was time to stop, she said, and she made it clear that she liked me more when I wasn't quite so bony. She reminded me of a mutual friend who had lost so much weight that it had started to show in his hollow-cheeked face and sunken eyes, and she told me in no uncertain terms that I was in danger of heading the same way. I looked in the mirror and agreed. For some people, knowing when to stop this diet can be just as important as recognising the need to start.

PORTION CONTROL

Greed is something my friend the Kitchen Guru and I have discussed at length—we both enjoy the button-popping feeling of being full. When we find something we like, we want more of it, even before we've finished the first helping. For some people, greed is hardwired into their personality, and coping with desire is complex. Part of it is wanting to feel full. Part of it is wanting more of a particular taste or texture—sugar, fat or a satisfying crunch. And part of it is simply habit.

As well as thinking carefully about the type of food on your plate, it is absolutely essential to think very carefully about how much you eat. There are a couple of really simple tricks to reduce portion size. First, slow down and chew your food for twice as long as you normally would. It takes concentration, but it really does help. Second, look at your plate or bowl and ask yourself if its contents are at most two-thirds of what you would normally put on a plate. If it's more than that, simply put some back. It's a primitive calculation, but it needs to be at the front of your mind as you consider portion sizes. For good measure, I banished large dinner plates and used smaller side plates for most meals. Empty space on a big dinner plate offers too much temptation.

Your mind may play tricks on you. There may be an indignant, instinctive response when you look at your reduced portion sizes. Your inner voice might ask, "Is that all I can have? I'll be hungry!" And dealing with hunger is an issue you must face head on if it comes up. There are numerous ways to handle it. My experience taught me to:

- Bulk up the low-carb vegetable content of main meals.

- Drink a large glass of water if hunger pangs start to bite.

- Snack on strawberries, raspberries or blueberries to satisfy the craving for sweet things.

- I chose not to skip breakfast, although there is a growing band of people (including some doctors and several of my close work colleagues) who believe that skipping breakfast is a useful way to undertake a short-term fast with encouraging results. It wasn't for me though.

- Slow down my eating.

I found it was useful to eat evening meals earlier rather than later. On the weekend, I would often eat as early as 6 p.m. Leaving at least three hours between the last meal of the day and going to bed also helped make me feel less listless and drowsy the following morning. But if you find yourself waking up unusually early, you may want to experiment with the time you eat your last meal. Some people on a calorie-restricted diet do need to eat a little later to avoid being ravenously hungry when they wake up. It's all a matter of personal choice.

I read a lot about the theory of "embracing hunger" as I prepared for this. I snorted disbelievingly at people who promoted the idea that embracing hunger is a good thing. Then something curious happened: I achieved a mid-morning high that became curiously compulsive. It wasn't exactly hunger; it was a mild euphoria. I'd find myself very alert and bouncing around the office, talking slightly too quickly and racing up the stairs like an enthusiastic Tigger. It didn't last past lunchtime, but it did become slightly addictive. It rarely came on in the mid-afternoon (the most dangerous period of the day for snacking for me), but as I experienced this mild euphoria, I started to understand and even enjoy what psychologists mean when they talk about embracing hunger.

I debated the issue of hunger with a colleague at work and had a sudden, if perhaps not very original, thought. We confuse hunger (by which I mean real hunger) with cravings. I've only been genuinely hungry a very few times on this diet, but I've had cravings almost every day, and it's easy to mistake the two. Hunger is your body telling you that you need to eat something, anything. But a craving is for something very particular and often something bad for you—a biscuit, a pastry or a bar of chocolate. Coping with cravings becomes a test of determination and willpower. I dealt with it by looking at the confectionery and bread counters and imagining great big boxes of diabetes pills and needles in place of the chocolate, breads and pastries. Crazy, perhaps, but it worked for me.

Eating out and snacking (particularly office snacking with birthday cakes and mid-afternoon "treats") are my Achilles heel. Snacking between meals needs to stop. At work, we have a "Filing Cabinet of Joy" in the middle of the office, laden with chocolate, muffins, biscuits, pastries and tins of sweets. Snacks help the office feel sociable, and they can be overpoweringly tempting, particularly as mid-afternoon fatigue sets in. With these cravings, I confess that I often failed as much as I succeeded.

One of my solutions was to bore my office colleagues relentlessly about my diet, and I could feel the harsh, baleful glares that came my way when I came hunting for snacks. My colleagues would stare me out as I descended on the biscuit barrel, and I am grateful to them for hiding them from me on numerous occasions, despite my petulance. One particularly ruthless colleague even took to calling me out publicly as I manoeuvred towards the biscuit barrel. 'Stop the diabetic!' she once shouted loudly to a shocked open-plan office. I owe her a debt of great gratitude.

SUGAR, SPICE, SALT AND SAUCES

Sugar, particularly refined sugar, is another thing that needs to go. Sweets, puddings, heaped teaspoons of sugar in tea and coffee, honey, jam, pastries, fruit juices, breakfast cereals, processed sauces, pre-prepared meals—the list goes on and on, and they all need to be banished. I swapped out real sugar in coffee for sweetener (many people advise against this), and in the last few weeks of the diet, I bought a sugar-replacement product containing xylitol that I used in very small quantities and only very rarely.

In the months before going on this diet, I'd tried some diabetic substitutes, such as sugar-free chocolate, and they were all horrible. They also contain sugar replacements that can play havoc with blood sugar levels and the digestive system; many have just as many calories as regular products, and they are absurdly expensive. It is possible to kick the sweet-tooth habit. It just takes time.

Some people will advise removing fruit from the diet altogether, but not me. I did remove some higher-carb or high-sugar fruits, particularly those with a high GI. The GI of a food is a measure of how quickly sugar from the food enters the bloodstream. Foods are scored on a GI scale between one and one hundred; the higher the number, the more quickly sugar enters the bloodstream.

I had primarily opted to reduce sugars and carbs, so dried fruits of most kinds as well as oranges, mangoes, pineapple, melon and bananas were all out. Fresh dark fruits became my go-to choices and I got my fruit boosts from blackberries, blueberries, raspberries, strawberries and plums, which all make great snacks and desserts, but not in large quantities and not every day.

Sadly, grapes were off the list because they have 16g of carbs per 100g. That busts the 10g rule, and they also have a high GI score. Apples also, depressingly, break the 10g carb limit and moderately affect blood sugar levels since they contain sugar, but much of it is fructose. When fructose is consumed in a whole fruit, it has less of an effect on blood sugar levels. I couldn't live without apples, so I just broke my own 10g rule for apples and kept them in.

There are two recipes in this book that use dark chocolate in small quantities—the No-Bean Chilli (*see page 130*) and the Caponata *(see page 119)*. I fought with the Kitchen Guru about including this ingredient in these recipes, but each contains less than one small square per serving, and the taste benefit outweighed anything else. You could always leave them out if you're stronger than I am.

The other thing that needs to be moderated is salt. That doesn't mean that it needs to be cut out altogether, but foods (particularly processed foods, pre-prepared sauces and takeaways) with high salt content need to be restricted, not because doing so will affect blood glucose scores or contribute to weight loss, but because it can reduce the risk of complications that come along with high blood pressure and can help alleviate water retention. The majority of salt in most people's diet doesn't come from the pinch or two added to a recipe or the dash of soy sauce used to flavour a dish; it comes from processed, pre-packaged foods, including commercial jars of sauces and salad dressings and many ready-made meals, all of which need to be banished.

Many of the small tubs of dressing lurking in the corners of high-street lunchtime salad boxes are surprisingly calorie-laden. There are 345 calories in the UK's version of Pret a Manger's "Chef's Italian Salad" box, for example. It's delicious. This salad became a lunchtime staple for me for many weeks—a satisfying blend of chicken, roasted red (bell) peppers, tomatoes, salad leaves, olives and pistachios. The minuscule pot of dressing that comes with it, however, hides another whopping 230 calories. Throw the pot away and replace it with a generous drizzle of olive oil and a squeeze of lime. I countered the reduction in salt by ramping up the spice (chillis in particular) and lemon juice.

ALCOHOL

As friends and family members interrogated me about what I was doing with my diet, alcohol was often the biggest issue. There's no good way to say this, so I'll just say it: all alcohol is off limits for the first eight weeks of this regime—despite Banting's experience in the 19th century. In the third and fourth sections of the programme, alcohol can return sparingly, but it will still count badly against your daily calorie targets. By the time you get to week nine, you can reintroduce alcohol in very limited quantities. It's hard, but remember, it's only temporary.

I chose to reintroduce alcohol after the first eight weeks, but some things were out for the duration of this process. For example, all beers, ciders, stouts and lagers went away; I also banished cocktails with conventional mixers, such as gin and tonic, all syrup-based cocktails, Alco pops and anything made with fresh fruit juices. After the first eight weeks, wine was OK in limited quantities (but not sweet wines), as were pure spirits (mixed with soda water, lime or light mixers). I struggled very hard to find a cocktail that I could drink, so at the end of the recipe section I've included one single awesome recipe for a low-carb, no-sugar margarita that came back at the end of week eight. It's a small tribute to the moment when this all began. It is my go-to low-carb cocktail of choice, and even though it looks simple on the page, it took forever to get right.

SAMPLE WEEKLY MEAL PLAN

I've included 40 recipes at the back of this book. Some are quite elaborate, and many feature fish and seafood or other specialty foods. Many of these recipes won't work for everyone's day-to-day life—particularly during the week, when time is short. I hope the recipes are useful as inspiration for weekend meals or for special occasions, but for those who want a quicker, easier solution, here is an example of what I ate Monday to Friday, when time was short and I needed quick, easy, healthy food, or when I ate out with friends.

I made a habit of pre-preparing some food for the week every weekend. Knowing that there is something at home in the fridge or freezer helps with the temptation of taking the easy option and eating out regularly during the week. I chose to eat regularly three times a day: breakfast, lunch and dinner. I know people who have adopted a different routine and who skip breakfast with some success (particularly if they eat early the preceding evening). It is a form of intermittent fasting that works for some people, but it wasn't for me. For lunch, I chose to prepare a boxed lunch several times a week, and on other days, I became a regular customer of my local Pret a Manger, which offers a wide range of pre-prepared, low-carb boxed salads.

Breakfast

This is often the hardest meal of the day for many people who are used to sugary, carb-laden cereals or a quick croissant on the go.

- Full fat Greek yoghurt with fresh blueberries and raspberries
- Protein bread toast *(see page 81)* with cream cheese and ham
- 2-egg cheese omelette
- 2 scrambled eggs with avocado side salad
- Grilled sausage (find a variety without added breadcrumbs) and a poached egg

Lunch

- Pre-prepared chicken Caesar salad with crispy bacon and avocado
- Pre-prepared rare roast beef salad with baby spinach leaves and baby tomatoes
- Green bean and tuna salad with a hard-boiled egg and salad leaves
- A generous slice of homemade pre-prepared vegetable frittata
- Chicken soup without noodles

Dinner

- Stir-fried chicken with vegetables and chilli
- Grilled steak with garlic butter, green beans and a side salad
- Pan-fried salmon steak with a spinach and blue cheese salad
- Grilled lamb chops with roasted Mediterranean vegeatables
- No-Bean Chilli *(see page 130)* made in advance in bulk and frozen served with guacamole, sour cream and a leafy green salad

EXERCISE

The other thing that I decided needed to start in week one—and last for the entire period and beyond—was a modest exercise regime. I'm no exercise freak. I've joined gyms and never gone. I've hired trainers and skipped appointments. Exercise is up there with visits to the dentist in my list of all-time least-favourite activities.

The very strict advice from the Newcastle study was not to increase exercise levels during the weight-loss period, because "subconscious compensatory eating will make weight loss very difficult." It suited me down to the ground to follow this advice, though I did start a brisk walking regime immediately. I was excessively sedentary—not just a little bit lazy, but really very idle indeed. I concluded that I needed to achieve 10,000 steps a day, the default goal of most fitness trackers. This is another discussion you have to have with your medical advisor; together, you need to decide the right level of daily exercise for you.

Not all steps are equal. A slow dawdle won't cut it. The goal is 10,000 brisk steps. Imagine you're late for a meeting—that's brisk. Or walk to your favourite beat; anything over 120 beats per minute counts. That includes many ABBA songs, I was pleased to discover. Check out songbpm.com[30] for your favourite tracks. It needs to become a daily habit, even on weekends, when it's hardest to achieve. The closest station to where I live is less than a two-minute walk away, so I chose to walk to the next closest, which is around 13 minutes away. I walk there and back, every day—even on weekends. Briskly.

I trained myself to get off the bus at least two stops earlier than I normally would. I would walk to the supermarket, rather than use the car. I used the stairs at work, rather than the lift, and took them two steps at a time. I spent 10 minutes of my lunch break walking briskly, even if I had no specific destination in mind. And if when I got home at night I hadn't completed the 10,000-step goal, I'd turn around and walk until I had. I found it to be an essential part of this regime. It becomes very important towards the end of the plan, and it will be just as important as you start to focus on maintenance.

To burn fat through exercise requires a significant investment of time and commitment. Walking will certainly help, but it may not be enough to maintain a healthy lifestyle as you go through this diet. Exercise also helps regulate blood glucose levels—another important reason to get off the sofa or get off the bus one stop earlier than you normally would. And if fasting blood glucose levels fluctuate unexpectedly, a light regular exercise regime can help stabilise the scores.

---

30 https://songbpm.com

Brisk walking, although it helps, doesn't really raise the heartbeat sufficiently or increase aerobic capacity enough to make a significant impact. Six weeks into the diet I added a simple home-based cardio workout to my walking target to increase my stamina. A friend gave me a sequence of easy routines that I had to do every day. I had no interest in developing any muscles; I simply wanted a short, high-intensity exercise routine that I could do at home each morning. My arms, core and shoulders needed strengthening, and my stamina needed to increase. A simple combination of stretches, a few weights and a sequence of sit-ups and push-ups, repeated three times with short breaks to allow my body to recover between sequences, did the trick.

I resented the idea of spending money on exercise equipment, so I salvaged two large granite bricks from the garden to use as improvised dumbbells. I was sceptical, but within three weeks it got easier, then it got much easier. And one day I flexed my upper arm and there were tiny muscles on both sides of the upper arm. Within six weeks, they were big enough to see through the slightly skinnier T-shirts I'd started wearing. And by the end of three months, I had both stomach and upper-arm muscles and much stronger shoulders. I'm never going to be ripped. A six-pack will never appear; I simply don't have the dedication. But it was a dramatic transformation, and it was very worthwhile.

Sleep is the other key issue in this regime. I curtailed some elements of my social life—not least because of the temptations and challenges of eating out and sitting in bars while friends snaffle crisps and salty snacks, drink cocktails and munch on burgers. Cutting back on my social life left me with more time on my hands at home. The consequence was that I started going to bed earlier than I had for much of my adult life. I tried to leave at least three hours after eating the last meal of the day before going to bed, which meant that I was often in bed by 10 p.m. and rarely after 10:30 p.m. On weekends, I often went to bed half an hour earlier.

Sticking to a regular sleeping routine is important. For me, the connection between a low-carb diet and waking up early is direct and immediate. On a low-carb regime, I always wake up earlier and have more energy first thing in the morning. If I bust the diet and demolish an entire pizza or burger, I see an immediate effect the following morning. I wake up much later, feeling very listless and wanting to stay in bed. But midway through this process, I had an overwhelming urge to get up as soon as I woke up—my body was telling me to get active in the early morning. It actually took a conscious effort to stay in bed if I woke up very early. To the consternation of my close friends, I even bought a pair of running shoes and started a light run every third morning as the sun came up over the suburbs of west London. I aimed for at least seven hours of good-quality sleep a night[31].

OTHER PEOPLE

I had some amazing support from the people around me as I did this. My friends and colleagues were limitless in their encouragement as they put up with my obsession.

Not everyone was kind. Someone asked me in a meeting if my breath smelled bad while I was on the diet. A thoughtless neighbour smiled through gritted teeth and told me she'd seen many people drop weight like this, but everyone had piled it back on eventually. Shifting the conversation to the subject of reversing a diabetes diagnosis, rather than talking about weight loss, generally stopped people when they were being unkind. Other people tipped their head to one side, grimaced sympathetically and asked in hushed tones if I was ill. I told them I had been, but I was hopefully getting better, which was true—just not in the way they meant.

My strong advice is to talk to everyone about what you're doing— friends, family, and colleagues—as it helps provide an incentive to

---

31 https://www.nhs.uk/oneyou/sleep#xowX82yBfxO6ZWDm.97

keep it up. The dinner party invitations might become a little more infrequent, but personally, I didn't mind for a while. It helped keep temptation at bay.

CLOTHES

I went through three entire wardrobes. For a while, I had my big clothes, mostly 2XL. When they started to look a bit baggy, I invested in some cheap mid-range clothes sized XL and L. And now I have my new wardrobe—mostly M. I was told to put all my big clothes in a box and mark "Richard's Fat Clothes" on it with a big red pen to serve as a reminder of how I used to be. Water retention may skew the weigh-ins, but your wardrobe will speak to you loudly as your body changes shape.

The high-street chains that were previously off limits, as they had no clothes in my size, became my new playgrounds. For the first time in my life, I visited stores that stocked sportswear. I'm tall with a long torso and quite broad shoulders, so not all medium-size clothes are for me, but many are. I took to wearing tight, stretchy polo shirts and clingy breathable Lycra, often for effect rather than for comfort. The first time I wore a skinny, roll-neck sweater to work, I was channelling Steve Jobs. It was the first time someone turned to me and told me I was too thin.

An unexpected downside of my diet was a stupid, vanity-inspired, self-inflicted side effect. To complete the transformation, I started wearing skinny jeans with very tight belts. *Meralgia paresthetica* is a nerve condition characterised by tingling, numbness and a sudden stabbing, burning pain in the outer part of your front thigh caused by compression of a nerve that supplies sensation to the upper leg. It can be caused by excessively tight clothes—in my case, by a ridiculously tight belt. It was entirely my own doing; I really didn't need a tight belt to show off my new 32-inch waist. It was a painful lesson in vanity.

SUMMARY

This plan relies on dramatically reducing carbohydrates, reducing calories for a limited period of time, removing sugars, modestly increasing exercise levels and ensuring that you stay hydrated.

- **Carbohydrates:** We all need carbohydrates to function, but this low-carb plan focuses on foods that contain less than 10g of carbs per 100g, including meat, fish, seafood, full-fat natural dairy products, natural oils and fats, above-the-ground vegetables and some fruits. All flour-based products, bread, cakes, pastry, biscuits and pasta, as well as rice and potatoes, are out.

- **Sugars:** Our diets are laden with processed sugars. Confectionery is off the list, as are many sauce-based takeaways, bottled pre-prepared sauces, fruit juices, honey products and breakfast cereals. I also put aside certain fruits, such as melon, pineapple, mango and bananas. All of these can come back later, but for the duration of this plan I avoided them and replaced them with fresh blueberries, blackberries, raspberries and strawberries.

- **Calories:** I chose to combine a low-carb approach with reducing calories for a limited period. The calorie reduction was progressively less ruthless over time, as it was greater at the beginning of the plan than at the end. Attempting to maintain weight loss over a long period of time by calorie reduction alone is likely to be a fruitless exercise, as the body will eventually adapt to the reduced calorie intake.

- **Exercise:** An important part of this regime for me was to become less sedentary. I followed a very simple rule that involved at least 30 minutes of brisk walking every day, including weekends. If you commit to adding a very short additional exercise routine that includes raising your heartbeat for a limited period of time through gentle jogging or swimming three times a week, the benefits will start to show in a few short weeks.

- **Water:** Staying hydrated was an equally important issue for me. Before I started this programme, I drank very little water, but it helped me feel full when I was feeling hungry and counteracted the digestion problems that can come with a low-carb diet.

It is very important to stay in touch with your doctor or a nutritionist during this programme. There can be some very significant risks associated with changing your diet, and for some people, these risks can be far greater than the original diabetes diagnosis itself. Seek medical advice before you embark on this regime and as you go through it, and do not change your medications without talking to your doctor first.

AFTER WEEK 16

There's no real hard end to this regime. It just fades into a newly modified real life with a reduced appetite for carbs and sugars and an aversion to processed foods. If your experience is anything like mine, the bulk of the weight loss will happen during the start and middle of the programme, and after three or four months, it's likely that the weight-loss curve will simply flatten out. There might be something of a bounce at the end. Set yourself an upper limit, and if you go over it, it's important for long-term maintenance to repeat a shorter version of the programme for a few weeks to bring yourself back within range.

And as you return to a normal calorie intake, you may well find that your tastes have changed. Maintaining a calorific deficit won't work for long-term maintenance, but restricting carbs and sugars may need to stay with you for a long time. The controversy over long-term low-carb diets doesn't show any sign of abating. In 2018, a report[32] based on observational studies rather than clinical trials from Brigham and Women's Hospital in Boston reported that low-carb diets might be associated with shorter overall life spans in the long term. The study found that people who ate a moderate amount of carbohydrates had a life expectancy four years longer than those on a low-carb diet. The regime I am describing in this book is based on my own short-term experience to promote sufficient weight loss to reverse diabetes. It is

32 http://uk.businessinsider.com/amount-of-carbs-to-eat-for-a-long-life-2018-8

not a manifesto for a lifelong commitment to a low-carb lifestyle. I chose to reintroduce carbs in limited quantities after I completed my weight loss, but this is a personal choice, and I know several people who have chosen to maintain their commitment to low-carb long after they have vanquished their diabetes. The choice of what you do after this comes to an end is yours to be made in conjunction with your medical practitioner. I promised myself that when I reached my target weight, I'd reward myself by consuming an entire box of Viennese Whirls, but when the moment came, I simply didn't want them.

To this day, I don't really eat potatoes, rice or pasta in any great quantities. Bread came back in a limited way and only in the mornings, really. I rarely have it at lunchtime and never in the evenings. I found I had lost my taste for quick-fix sweet treats. And I knew that I needed to continue with a modest exercise regime.

Five months after starting this regime, I booked in for a set of blood tests. As I walked into the surgery, my diabetes nurse summoned up my records. She scanned me up and down. "Are you diabetic?" she asked as the computer whirred into life and brought up my records. "I hope not!" I said. She looked at me with a wry, broad smile as she studied my records. I told her what I'd done and showed her some pictures on my iPhone. She was silent for a few seconds; then, she asked if the old pictures were really me.

A week later, I called for the results. My doctor went through the scores. It was a moment I had imagined for a long time. A close friend had counselled me to prepare for disappointing news—he asked what my reaction would be if my scores still defined me as diabetic, despite the weight loss. It doesn't work for everyone, he gently reminded me. I was sanguine. I concluded that my overall health would be better, whichever way the results went.

The results were comfortably below the threshold that defined me as a diabetic. I wasn't even pre-diabetic. We talked for a while and looked through my scores from the last few years. I expected to feel a bit emotional and, of course, I was happy, but something inside me knew what I was going to hear. It all felt a little anticlimactic. I just felt normal, and I'd felt normal for several weeks at that point.

Diabetic remission doesn't just arrive one day with a single set of results—particularly if someone is still taking meds. I was told to come off the cholesterol meds straight away. But there was a pause when it came to a discussion about the diabetes medicine. In clinical settings, when people undertake this regime under close medical supervision, diabetic medication is removed very early on, as some meds can interact very dangerously with reduced carb regimes. But my doctor said that this was a new situation for her, and she wanted to make some calls. I decided to take matters into my own hands. Three weeks after my scores came in, I simply stopped taking the pills. I suggest you think extremely carefully before you do the same, and definitely talk to your doctor before you do anything quite so rash.

Months came and went. The computer system continued to pump out letters asking me to come in for foot and blood tests. I decided to wait for a while before I took another test—again, not something that I would recommend. Nine months later, I checked in again and went through another full diabetic review. My feet were examined, and the bloods were drained. Truthfully, I was more anxious about this moment than I had been nine months earlier, as I was no longer on medication. I wondered if perhaps the meds had actually helped me achieve such low scores the previous summer.

My nurse asked me what tablets I was taking. When I told her I had come off everything, she became concerned. "Why have you done this?" she asked. "Why haven't we been testing you more regularly?" I didn't really have an answer. It was Easter weekend, almost exactly six years since my vision had collapsed so dramatically. As I waited for the results over the holiday weekend, I looked at the shelves piled high with Easter eggs and chocolates and walked past them without wanting to tempt fate. Next year, perhaps? I wanted the next scores to be at least the same as, or perhaps better than, the scores I had achieved nine months earlier.

My HbA1c (the test used to reflect average blood glucose levels over the preceding eight to twelve weeks) had improved. I was 5.6 percent (38mmol/mol). It had stabilised well below the diabetic threshold of 6.5 percent (48mmol/mol)—not even pre-diabetic. It was a surprise, as I hadn't been entirely angelic in the intervening nine months. I was absolutely sure that my occasional transgressions would be picked up by the HbA1C test, but it was all fine.

Rather more surprising was my fasting blood glucose (the test that measures blood glucose control). I had been ruthless in the week leading up to the test. The result, 6.4mmol/l (115.2mg/dL), was also below the 7mmol/l (126mg/dL) that would classify me as diabetic, but it wasn't far off. I very much wanted it to be lower.

I immediately interpreted it as a warning sign that I could be at risk for a new type 2 diagnosis at some point in the future. A single fasting blood glucose score of this level on its own doesn't confirm a pre-diabetic diagnosis, and I was told there was no need for medication, but I was firmly advised that I needed to maintain a healthy diet, get more exercise, limit my alcohol consumption, drink less coffee, sleep properly and finally quit smoking.

Although I had lost more than thirty kilos, had changed my diet and looks and had successfully come off all medications without any significant side effects, it just wasn't quite as perfect as I had wanted it to be. I was cross—furious, actually. I didn't like or trust the result. I promptly went out and bought myself a blood glucose monitor and, for the first time in my life, I self-tested every morning for two months. I recommitted myself to a gentle exercise regime, cut back on my daily coffee intake, banished alcohol during the week, threw away the marmalade and stopped eating croissants.

I did fasting blood glucose tests every day for two months. Measuring daily blood glucose became an incredibly useful exercise. In addition to being able to see a direct relationship between blood glucose levels and the sugars and carbs I consumed, I also discovered that my fasting blood glucose scores could also be affected by a wide range of other things, including dehydration, stress or other illnesses, too much caffeine or alcohol, too little exercise, long-haul flights or a poor sleep regime.

Within three days, my score had dropped to 5.1mmol (91.8mg/dL). A week later, it was 4.7mmol (84.6mg/dL), well below even a pre-diabetic threshold. Over the following sixty days, it averaged 5.3mmol (95.4mg/dL)—exactly the same non-diabetic score I'd achieved nine months earlier, while I was still on the meds.

With some lapses here and there, I'd generally stayed on a pretty low-carb regime since coming off the meds. People on a long-term low-carb diet can sometimes experience an early morning high followed by a decline throughout the day. It's not an indicator of a blood sugar problem; instead, it is an adaptation the body makes as it uses fat as fuel. The science behind unexpected variations in fasting blood scores on a low carb diet is complex and beyond me, but when I questioned it, I was reassured that it's completely normal.

Nevertheless, the month of daily blood tests allowed me to experiment in order to find my ultimate daily meal plan. In a slightly compulsive experiment over four consecutive weekends, I decided to eat exactly the same thing each Sunday to see how consistently I could control my fasting blood scores. It needed to be food that I really liked, it needed to be satisfying and nutritious and it needed to include alcohol. In addition to drinking at least 2½ litres of water and walking at least 10,000 steps, my ideal daily Sunday regime was:

- BREAKFAST: Two pieces of protein bread toast (*see page 81*) with full-fat cream cheese and Parma ham, a crunchy green apple and two cups of strong coffee with full-fat milk.

- LUNCH: A small bowl of salted almonds and a glass of dry white wine followed by a two-egg Gruyère cheese omelette with a side of fried bacon and a fine green bean salad with crumbled feta, cherry tomatoes and black olives.

- DINNER: A bowl of vodka gazpacho soup with crème fraîche or full-fat sour cream followed by a crab, chilli and spring onion salad in gem lettuce cups and a shrimp and avocado side salad, and for dessert, a small bowl of full-fat Greek yoghurt topped with a handful of strawberries and blueberries and toasted pecans.

That's roughly 1,750 calories, 54g of carbs, 112g of protein and 72g of fat. It consistently produced a fasting blood glucose score the next day between 4.8mmol (86.4mg/dL) and 5.2mmol (93.6mg/dL).

My full scores over the six-year period were:

HbA1c

Diabetes:	*6.5% (48mmol/mol) or higher*
Pre-diabetes:	*5.7%–6.4% (39mmol/mol–46.4mmol/mol)*
Normal:	*below 5.7% (39mmol/mol)*
March 2012	14.9% (139mmol/mol)
April 2012	10.5% (91mmol/mol)
June 2012	6.8% (51mmol/mol)
March 2014	6% (42mmol/mol)
January 2017*	6.7% (50mmol/mol)
August 2017**	5.7% (39mmol/mol)
April 2018	5.6% (38mmol/mol)

Fasting blood glucose

Diabetes:	*7mmol/L or higher (126mg/dL)*
Pre-diabetes:	*5.5mmol/L–6.9mmol/L (100mg/dL–125mg/dL)*
Normal:	*below 5.5mmol/L (100mg/dL)*
March 2012	23mmol (414mg/dL)
April 2012	7.4mmol (133.2mg/dL)
June 2012	7.5mmol (135mg/dL)
March 2014	7.6mmol (136.8mg/dL)
January 2017*	9.1mmol (163.8mg/dL)
August 2017**	5.3mmol (95.4mg/dL)
March 2018	6.4mmol (115.2mg/dL)
April/May 2018***	5.3mmol (95.4mg/dL)

* Start of diet
** Weight loss target achieved/end of medications
*** 60-day FBG average

It was over. Except it's never quite over—not really. My scores are towards the upper end of a non–pre-diabetic range, and the effective control of body fat, sugar consumption, carbs and exercise levels will be all-important in the years ahead. I know now that, in itself, a single fasting blood glucose score isn't the important marker. HbA1c is the key signifier of diabetes, along with unexplained weight loss, increased hunger and excessive thirst. And, like anyone of my age, my lipids and cholesterol levels will need to be checked, and my HbA1c will be regularly monitored. If it does ever start to creep back up, I'll be back into a routine of foot exams, boxes of pills and automated letters. But that's not happening. For now, I'm done.

REMISSION

The DiRECT trial has a few wise words about post-remission maintenance—it tells us that it is the hardest part of the process,[33] as if everything up to this moment hasn't been tricky enough. It advises people to seek help from a local nutritionist to come up with strategies for holidays and social occasions in order to avoid regaining weight. And if you do start to put weight back on, it adds, it is essential to spot it right away and act quickly to minimise the regain. Weigh yourself at least weekly, and if your weight rises by 2kg or more, you need to put together an urgent strategy to bring it back down again—one that includes exercise.

Maintaining stability after diabetic remission is, as I have discovered, a complex subject. I'm only at the very beginning of this part of the journey. For me, it comes down to a careful balance between providing my body with sufficient nutrients (and calories) to function efficiently; maintaining a commitment to consume fewer carbs, no refined sugars and no processed foods; enjoying all the benefits of exercise; and a little intermittent fasting—the details of this are destined for a future publication.

There are very few studies on what happens in the long term after diabetic remission. But a tantalising glimpse of the future lies in a quotation from Professor Taylor, who announced: "The study also answered the question that people often ask me—if I lose the weight and keep the weight off, will I stay free of diabetes? The simple answer is yes! Interestingly, even though all our volunteers remained obese or overweight, the fat did not drift back to clog up the pancreas."[34]

The difference between "remission" and "cure" when it comes to type 2 diabetes is a hotly contested subject, and many medical

---

33 http://www.directclinicaltrial.org.uk/Documents/Patient%20Info%20Website%20Feb%202018.pdf

34 http://www.ncl.ac.uk/press/articles/archive/2016/03/profroytaylordiabetesresearch/

professionals question whether it is ever accurate to say that a chronic illness is technically "cured". For many in prolonged diabetic remission, there is a self-evident predisposition for symptoms to return without an enduring long-term commitment to a permanently changed lifestyle.

Almost exactly a year after coming off all medications, a letter arrived from the NHS inviting me to attend an annual diabetic eye test. The date and time had been decided by the computer, and I was to call only if I couldn't attend. Multiple text messages and automated phone calls followed. I called and explained that I was in remission, that I was no longer taking any pills with my doctor's blessing. I told them that the appointment could be used for someone in greater need.

The lady on the telephone paused. I could hear pages being thumbed. It seemed as though she was looking for the right answer from a script.

"'Diabetes is a lifelong condition…'" she started to say.

"Stop!" I said, quietly. "It isn't."

She paused and tried again. "Diabetes will always be with you."

It felt as though the medical profession was questioning what I had done. I was told that if I refused the appointment, my doctor would be told about my lack of compliance. We agreed to disagree.

An influential paper on this subject published in September 2017[35] makes the point that it's important to achieve consensus on an appropriate classification system for diabetic remission, because a diabetes diagnosis can affect so many parts of our lives. There can be negative consequences for insurance premiums (in particular, for life and travel insurance[36]); for driving[37]; and in employment practices.

35 http://www.directclinicaltrial.org.uk/Pubfiles/Beating%20Diabetes%20McCombie%202017%20bmj.j4030.full.pdf
36 https://www.diabetes.org.uk/how_we_help/financial_services/travel_insurance
37 https://www.gov.uk/diabetes-driving

In a few well-publicised cases, people have felt that they have been discriminated against at work because of a diabetes diagnosis[38].

Different studies have proposed different definitions of remission. One of these definitions is a healthy-range blood glucose with "an HbA1c below 6.5 percent (48mmol/mol) after 12 months, with at least two months without any type 2 diabetes medication."[36] An earlier study proposed: "Complete remission is a return to 'normal' measures of glucose metabolism (HbA1c in the normal range, fasting glucose <100mg/dL [5.6mmol/L]) of at least one year's duration in the absence of active pharmacologic therapy or on-going procedures."[36]

Whatever the future definition turns out to be, the same paper, which was published by the American Diabetes Association in 2009, cannily references the way many patients themselves actually see remission: "...terminology such as 'prolonged remission' is probably less satisfactory to patients than use of the more hopeful and definitive term 'cure.'"

I'm happy to leave the terminological discussion to the experts. I use the word *conquer*. That's good enough for me.

---

38 http://diabetestimes.co.uk/diabetes-uk-survey-reveals-discrimination-at-work/

THE RECIPES

The recipes here are mostly designed for two people. Some are very simple. Others take a little more effort.

There's a great deal of seafood here, particularly in the starter section. I'm sorry if fish isn't your thing, but I found that it worked wonders. It's a low-carb superfood, in my opinion. Some of the recipes appear similar at first glance—the tuna laab (*see page 89*), the seafood stacks (*see page 83 and 90*) or the tuna poke (*see page 109*), for instance—but the subtle variations in flavour and texture are significant. As my palate started to recognise the differences, the dishes became evermore complex and nuanced in their detail.

Many of the Asian and Japanese-inspired recipes, particularly in the starter section, also call for raw seafood. There's a big health warning here: any raw seafood dish (even if it's marinated in citrus) needs to use the freshest possible fish—straight from the fishmonger, not frozen and not wrapped in plastic on the supermarket shelves. Tell your fishmonger that you'll be eating it raw, and seek advice if you are unsure about the source or how fresh it is. If you don't like raw fish, you can substitute hot-smoked or canned varieties for many of these dishes, although they don't carry the same flavour. I know some people who use canned tuna in the tuna laab (*see page 89*), for example, but I don't advise it. And please look for a sustainable fish mark when you buy seafood.

There are one or two cheats that were added to the roster as my calorie restriction got less severe; even rice (in very small quantities) can make a very brief reappearance later in the regime. One recipe here (*see page 89*) calls for a small amount of toasted rice. I've included it in the book because it is just so delicious.

The Kitchen Guru's contributions to these recipes have been inestimable. Many of the main-course recipes are hers, although she was kind enough to let me interfere with them. She introduced me to the idea of putting pears in caponata (I use them very sparingly), and she also suggested very imaginative swaps in many of the accompanying side dishes. I'm greatly in her debt for her imagination, her depth of knowledge and her unswerving support through this regime. I am also grateful to the many chefs I have met throughout Europe and Asia who have generously allowed me to use and adapt their recipes.

The calorie and carb values of each recipe are only approximate and will vary according to each one's original ingredients, portion sizes and cooking methods. I used a great online recipe analysis tool[39] to calculate the values, but it isn't 100 percent accurate. Ingredients will vary from country to country, so the counts are only indicative. I've only included calorie and carbohydrate values here, but you can get the full nutritional values by pasting the ingredient list into any online recipe analyser.

Although it appears at first glance that some of the recipes bust the 10g carb rule, remember that the rule is about 10g of carbs per 100g serving—or 10 percent—so a 200g serving can have 20g of carbs on this plan. At the same time, remember that on this plan, carb reduction and temporary calorie reduction go hand in hand, so be modest with your portion sizes.

---

39 https://happyforks.com/analyzer

Breakfast can be a struggle. Many of us are programmed to eat carbs, cereals and sugars for breakfast, and finding something I liked for breakfast became a major challenge. It's quick and easy to grab a croissant or a fresh pastry, to toast some bread or to wolf down a bowl of cereal, but none of these things are allowed on this diet.

After weeks of trying and failing to bake my own almond bread and experimenting with coconut flour, I fell upon a product called protein bread from a local London bakery called the Bread Shop. They currently have only five stores in London, but they do mail order[40] if you can stand the delivery charges. The Bread Shop's protein bread has 24 percent protein and only 8 percent carbohydrates, and it claims to be rich in amino acids, high in fibre and omega 3. It also toasts brilliantly and freezes well.

Many supermarket varieties of protein bread simply have protein added to them. Be warned: these can score as high as other breads on the carb scale. But the Bread Shop's protein product is a revelation. There is also one version of a protein-bread mix made in Australia by the Protein Bread Company[41] that boasts 95 percent fewer carbs than regular bread. I'm told that it tastes delicious, but sadly, they currently only ship to Australia, New Zealand and the US.

I was fascinated to read about a breakfast alternative popular with many type 2 online groups, Bulletproof Coffee. Largely unknown in the UK, Bulletproof Coffee is the brainchild of Dave Asprey, a Silicon Valley tech entrepreneur who says he was inspired by the yak-butter tea he found while travelling in Tibet in 2004. It's a dense combination of coffee, two tablespoons of grass-fed unsalted butter and a product called Brain Octane Oil[42]. It has since spawned an entire Bulletproof diet. I'm told that Brain Octane Oil is 100 percent pure

---

40 http://www.breadshop.co.uk/buyonline/Product-Protein-Bread_95.aspx
41 https://theproteinbreadco.com.au/shop/protein-bread-mix/
42 https://www.theguardian.com/lifeandstyle/2017/may/14/
bulletproof-coffee-dave-asprey-eat-healthy-exercise-interview

coconut oil, cleaned with activated charcoal and refined using only heat, water, and pressure[43]. Some people supercharge it with additional coconut oil, although Dave disapproves of this practice. Bulletproof has many enthusiastic type-2 champions, but it's not for me. I've been teased once too often by my friends for drizzling yak's milk on stuff; although I've never actually drizzled yak's milk on anything personally, I can't bring myself to fulfil the cliché.

My own, more primitive breakfast solution was to swap between full-fat Greek yoghurt with fresh berries and a small helping of grain-free granola or raw nuts (almonds, walnuts, toasted pecans or hazelnuts) on day 1, cooked eggs on day 2 and toasted protein bread with cream cheese and Parma ham on day 3. Then, I'd repeat the sequence. It's a challenge to set aside the time to cook eggs every third day and overcome the morning cravings for carbs, but stick with it. Believe me, after a while, the cravings for Cocoa Krispies (87g of carbs per 100g), cornflakes (84g of carbs per 100g) and toast (50g to 60g of carbs per 100g) will eventually subside.

---

43 https://www.bulletproof.com/review/product/list/id/490/?p=55

STARTERS, SOUPS, SNACKS AND SALADS

CRAB, SPRING ONION, RADISH AND TOMATO STACKS

Fresh, spicy and refreshing, these simple stacks need to be made an hour or two before serving and they benefit from being chilled in the fridge. You will need four (8cm/3¼-in) food rings for this recipe, which can be found online or at any good kitchenware store.

Serves 2
Approximately 300 calories/8g total carbs per serving

100g/3½ oz picked white crab meat
Juice of ½ lemon
½ bunch spring onions (scallions), finely sliced
½ red chilli, very finely chopped
½ tbsp full-fat mayonnaise or Greek yoghurt
Sea salt and freshly ground black pepper
200g/7 oz ripe cherry tomatoes, thinly sliced
200g/7 oz radishes, finely sliced
Lamb's lettuce or rocket (arugula) salad, to serve
Olive oil and additional lemon juice, to drizzle over

Set 1 tbsp of the crab meat aside to use as a decoration at the end, then combine the rest with the juice of ½ lemon, spring onions (scallions), chilli, and mayonnaise or yoghurt. Stir to combine and season to taste.

Place an 8cm/3¼-in food ring in the centre of a serving plate and lay a thin layer of tomatoes at its base, then cover with 1 tbsp of the crab mixture, levelling it out into an even layer. Top with a layer of radish, then add another layer of crab. Repeat the layers until you reach the top of the ring, ensuring that the final layer is tomato. Without removing the ring, grind a little of the black pepper over the top layer and then press down on the stack with a small jar or weight that fits inside the ring to compress the layers. Repeat this process with the remaining three stacks. Transfer the stacks to the fridge with the rings and jars intact for a couple of hours to firm up—a little bit of juice may seep out while the stacks are chilling, but this can easily be mopped up before serving.

To serve, carefully remove the rings from the stacks by holding the jar in place and gently pulling up on the ring, put 2 stacks on each plate. Surround the exposed stacks with lamb's lettuce or rocket (arugula) leaves, lightly dressed with the additional lemon juice and olive oil. Top each stack with a little of the reserved crab, then top with a final grind of the black pepper and a drizzle of the additional lemon juice. Serve immediately.

Cook's tip: You can use other raw salad vegetables as a layer in these stacks: cucumber, very thinly sliced celery, diced avocado tossed in a little lemon juice, or even thinly sliced white onion. For an extra layer of creaminess, I sometimes like to add a layer of guacamole to the middle of the stack.

MUSSEL AND SPRING ONION SOUP

This recipe is a cheat's version of the classic moules mariniere *made using boxed mussels, which are available in many supermarkets. If you want to do it from scratch, buy mussels from local fishmongers and*

*then add them to the remaining ingredients in this recipe. And if you
don't want the trouble of shelling the mussels yourself, pre-cooked mussels are often available from the fish counter, although cooking them
without their shells will result in some loss of flavour.*

Serves 2 as a starter or 1 as a main course
Approximately 350 calories/15g total carbs per serving

- 1 tbsp olive oil
- ½ onion, finely chopped
- ½ carrot, finely diced
- ½ stick celery, finely chopped
- ½ red chilli, very finely chopped (optional; use a red birds-eye if you like spice)
- Sea salt and freshly ground black pepper
- 1 × 500g/1 lb 2 oz box shell-on, boil-in-the-bag mussels
- 125mL/4 fl oz/generous ½ cup white wine
- 125mL/4 fl oz/generous ½ cup vegetable bouillon stock made with low-salt organic Swiss vegetable stock
- 1 small knob butter
- 125mL/4 fl oz/generous ½ cup single (pouring) cream (half and half)
- 4 spring onions (scallions), roughly chopped
- Small squeeze of lemon juice
- 1 tsp chopped chives, to garnish

Place the oil in a shallow frying pan over medium heat. Once hot,
add the onion, carrot, celery and chilli, if using, and season with the
salt and black pepper. Cook, stirring, until the onion is translucent,
but not browned. It's OK for the carrots to retain some crunch, as
this adds texture to the finished dish. Set aside.

Cook the mussels according to the package instructions and then
remove them from their shells. Drain but reserve the cooking liquor.

Return the carrot and celery mixture to high heat and then add the
wine, stock, reserved cooking liquor from the mussels and butter.
Bring to a boil and cook rapidly until the liquid has reduced by a

third and started to thicken. Remove from the heat, then immediately stir in the mussels, single cream, spring onions (scallions) and the lemon juice and stir to combine. Divide the mixture between serving bowls and serve hot, garnished with the chives.

VODKA GAZPACHO WITH PARMESAN CRISPS

This is a great recipe to pull out of the bag at dinner parties, as it looks impressive but is actually incredibly simple. The Parmesan crisps add the satisfying crunch that people on low-carb diets often crave. Gazpacho recipes provoke fierce debate. This fiery recipe isn't authentic, but it is delicious, especially when served ice cold in shot glasses on a hot summer's day.

Serves 6
Approximately 100 calories/6g total carbs per serving (excluding the Parmesan crisps)

400g/14 oz tomatoes on the vine, roughly chopped
1 small red (bell) pepper, roughly chopped
½ cucumber, peeled and roughly chopped, plus extra, to serve
2 spring onions (scallions), chopped
½ red onion, chopped
1 large garlic clove, crushed
1 small red chilli, chopped
35mL/1¼ fl oz (1 generous shot) vodka
20mL/¾ fl oz olive oil
1 tsp sherry vinegar
1 tsp lemon juice
Dash Worcestershire sauce
Sea salt and freshly ground black pepper
Generous chunk Parmesan cheese, very finely grated
1 tbsp chopped chives or chervil, to garnish
1 tbsp soured cream, to serve

Place the tomatoes, red pepper, ½ cucumber, spring onions (scallions), onion, garlic and chilli in a liquidiser (food processor) and blend until smooth. Transfer the mixture to a sieve (strainer) set over a bowl and push through with a wooden spoon to remove all the liquid. Once all the liquid has been removed, discard the vegetable pulp.

Add the vodka, olive oil, vinegar, lemon juice and Worcestershire sauce and stir to combine. Season generously and then taste and adjust the seasoning if necessary. Cover the bowl and then transfer to the fridge for several hours before serving (the soup should be served very cold).

When the soup is chilling, make the Parmesan crisps. Preheat the grill (broiler) to medium and line a baking sheet with parchment paper. Divide the Parmesan into 6 evenly spaced mounds on the prepared baking sheet and then place under the grill for 3–4 minutes, until melted to light-golden, bubbling rounds perforated with holes. You will need to keep on an eye on the crisps while they are cooking, as they can turn from golden to burnt in a very short space of time. Allow the crisps to cool completely and then transfer them to an airtight container until ready to use. Alternatively, for an extra bit of showmanship, you can shape the crisps into cigar shapes by rolling them around the round handle of a wooden spoon while still hot and sliding them off the handle as soon as they start to crisp up.

To serve the soup, fill 6 small shot glasses with gazpacho and top each with a little of the extra diced cucumber, some of the chives or chervil and a small blob of soured cream.

CLARIFIED CHILLED TOMATO SOUP

This is a bit of a show-off recipe. If you can get really ripe tomatoes at the height of summer, this recipe is delicious and refreshing. Be patient when waiting for the liquid to drip through, and don't be tempted to squeeze the muslin to speed up the process, as it will ruin your perfectly golden, clear soup.

Serves 4
Approximately 100 calories/15g total carbs per serving

2kg/4 lb 8 oz very ripe tomatoes, diced
1 stick celery, chopped
½ onion, finely chopped
½ fennel bulb, chopped
1 garlic clove, crushed
Handful fresh basil leaves, torn
1 sprig thyme
Generous dash Tabasco sauce
Sea salt
8 cherry tomatoes, quartered, to serve
4 spring onions (scallions), chopped, to serve
1 tbsp finely chopped chives, to garnish

Place the tomatoes, celery, onion, fennel, garlic, basil leaves, Tabasco sauce and thyme in a large, nonmetallic bowl and season generously with the salt. Cover and chill in the fridge for 8 hours or overnight to let the flavours mingle and develop.

Once chilled, transfer the mixture to a liquidiser (food processor) and blend until combined, but not completely smooth. Pour the mixture into a clean muslin cloth, bring up the four corners and tie securely at the top. Suspend the muslin over a large bowl and leave the mixture to drip through for at least 2 hours, or until the mixture has stopped dripping. Don't be tempted to squeeze the bag.

Once everything has dripped through, discard the contents of the muslin and transfer the liquid to the fridge, covered, until well chilled.

When ready to serve, divide the cherry tomatoes and spring onions between 6 bowls and ladle over the chilled soup. Garnish with the chives and serve immediately.

TUNA LAAB

I'm grateful to Noboru Fukushi, the owner of Tai by Red Snapper, one of the best restaurants on Koh Samui in the Gulf of Thailand, for his version of tuna laab (also called laap, larp, lahb or lab), an Isaan-inspired dish often made with ground and chilled pork or chicken. His is a chilled raw tuna version reinvented for the sushi generation. It is the only recipe in this book that uses a small amount of toasted white rice, but it's so good and the quantities are so modest that it's allowable. Sadly, laab simply doesn't work without the trademark crunchy toasted rice.

Serves 2
Approximately 180 calories/10g total carbs per serving

  1 heaped tbsp uncooked Thai sticky white rice
  1 (200g) fillet sushi-grade tuna, diced into 5-mm/¼-in cubes
  1 small red onion or shallot, finely chopped
  2 spring onions (scallions), finely chopped
  4 fresh mint leaves, finely chopped
  Juice of 1 lime
  1 tsp dried chilli flakes
  ½ tbsp fish sauce (nam pla)
  8 crispy Little Gem lettuce leaves taken from the middle of the lettuce head, to serve
  1 tsp toasted sesame seeds, to serve

In a small frying pan, dry-toast the raw uncooked Thai sticky rice over medium heat without any oil until it turns a beautiful golden brown, about 10 to 12 minutes. Grind the toasted rice in a food processor or mortar and pestle until it is the consistency of medium-fine breadcrumbs.

Place all the ingredients except the lettuce leaves and sesame seeds but including the ground rice into a bowl and stir to combine. Transfer to the fridge, covered, for 30 minutes to allow the flavours to develop. (If you have a taste for more spice, you can add a very finely chopped red birds-eye chilli.)

Once chilled, spoon the mixture into the lettuce leaf cups, scatter over the toasted sesame seeds and serve immediately.

Cook's tip: In North East Thailand and Laos, laab is often served with a small side plate of raw green (string) beans, finely shredded cabbage, water spinach and Thai basil, which are eaten at the same time for added flavour and texture

TUNA, AVOCADO, PLUM AND WASABI STACKS

This is a fruitier, spicier version of the previous stack with a fiery hit of wasabi. It's got a sweet and spicy heat and works perfectly as a summer starter and a final garnish of guacamole makes them deliciously soft and creamy.

Serves 4
Approximately 200 calories/18g total carbs per serving

   1 avocado, ripe but still firm
   1 tbsp lemon juice, plus extra, to drizzle over
   150g/5½ oz/⅔ cup natural yoghurt
   1 tsp wasabi paste
   Freshly ground black pepper
   1 (200 g) fillet sushi-grade tuna, finely diced
   2 ripe dark plums, finely diced
   Lamb's lettuce or rocket (arugula) salad, to serve
   Chilli oil, to drizzle over
   2 tsp salmon caviar, to serve
   Guacamole, to serve

Finely chop the flesh of the avocado and drizzle over the 1 tbsp of lemon juice to prevent it turning brown. Set aside.

Place 2 tsp of the yoghurt, the wasabi paste and the remaining lemon juice in a small bowl and stir to combine. Season generously with the black pepper and then taste and adjust the seasoning if necessary. Add the diced tuna to the yoghurt and wasabi mixture and stir to combine. Set aside.

Place a (8cm/3¼-in) food ring in the centre of a serving plate and lay a thin layer of avocado at its base. Cover with 1 tbsp of the tuna mixture, levelling it out into an even layer. Top with a layer of diced plum and then add another layer of tuna. Repeat the layers until you reach the top of the ring, ensuring that the final layer is tuna. Without removing the ring, press down on the stack with a small jar or weight that fits inside the ring to compress the layers. Repeat this process with the remaining three stacks. Transfer the stacks to the fridge with the rings and jars intact for an hour to firm up.

To serve, carefully remove the rings from the stacks by holding the jar in place and gently pulling up on the ring. Surround the exposed stacks with the lamb's lettuce or rocket (arugula) leaves, lightly dressed with lemon juice and chilli oil. Top each stack with ½ tsp of the salmon caviar followed by a small blob of the yoghurt or guacamole, a final grind of the black pepper and a drizzle of the lemon juice. Serve immediately.

Cook's tip: If you dislike raw fish, you can substitute layers of cooked prawns for the tuna (make sure the backs of the prawns are touching the inside edge of the ring for maximum effect when you take the mould off) and, for added bite, you could add layers of finely chopped spring onion (scallion) or very finely sliced celery.

SALMON CARPACCIO WITH SHAVED FENNEL, CELERY AND CHILLI OIL DRESSING

This recipe was given to me by one of my favourite restaurants in the Canary Islands—although I think it's originally an Italian recipe. The fennel adds a deliciously refreshing aniseed note. The salmon should be sliced so thinly at the end that it's translucent, and it should cover the entire serving plate in one wafer-thin layer.

Serves 2
Approximately 300 calories/6g total carbs per serving

  1 (200g) fillet sushi-grade salmon
  2 tbsp chilli oil
  Zest and juice of 1 lemon
  Small bunch fresh dill, finely chopped
  ¼ bulb fennel, finely sliced
  2 sticks celery, finely sliced
  1 tbsp miniature capers
  1 tbsp olive oil
  Sea salt and freshly ground black pepper
  2 tbsp salmon caviar, to serve

Place the salmon fillet, chilli oil, lemon zest and half the dill in a zip-lock bag. Seal and gently massage to combine the flavours. Place the bag in the fridge for up to 8 hours or overnight to allow the flavours to develop.

When you are almost ready to slice the salmon, place the fennel and celery in a bowl with half the lemon juice and a generous grind of the black pepper. Set aside.

Remove the salmon from the bag and wipe off any dill that is stuck to the surface. Place on a board and, using a very sharp knife, slice the salmon as thinly as possible, creating almost translucent slices. Place the salmon slices on a serving platter in 1 thin layer and then dress sparingly with the fennel and celery mixture, the olive oil, the remaining dill and the capers. Season with the salt and black pepper. Dot over some of the salmon caviar, add a final squeeze of the lemon juice and serve immediately.

Cook's tip: If you are struggling to slice the salmon to the required thinness, try placing the fillet in the freezer for 30 minutes to firm up before slicing.

SMOKED TROUT PÂTÉ WITH CELERY STICKS

A super-simple appetiser with a powerful crunch. When you stuff the mixture into the celery sticks, make sure it's piled generously on top, or serve it as a dip in a bowl for people to dive in themselves. Carrot batons, radishes or crisp spring onions (scallions) also work well if you are serving this as a dip.

Serves 4
Approximately 250 calories/9g total carbs per serving

  180g/6 oz/¾ cup full-fat cream cheese
  2 fillets smoked trout, skin removed
  Zest and juice of 1 lemon
  Small bunch chives, finely chopped
  ½ red chilli, finely chopped
  1 tbsp jarred "nonpareille" capers
  1 pinch cayenne pepper
  1 tbsp horseradish sauce or 1 tsp finely grated fresh horseradish
    (optional)
  6 sticks celery, cut into 2-inch pieces, to serve
  Sea salt and freshly ground black pepper

Place the cream cheese in a bowl and flake in the trout, keeping an eye out for any bones as you do. Using a fork, mash the cream cheese and fish together until almost smooth, but retaining some texture. Add the lemon zest and juice, chives, chilli, capers and cayenne pepper and horseradish, if using, and stir until well combined. Season to taste with the salt and black pepper. Transfer to the fridge, covered, for at least 1 hour.

Once chilled, spoon the pâté into the grooves of the celery sticks and use a knife to spread down their length. Serve immediately.

BRESAOLA, PARMESAN AND ROCKET ROLLS

This recipe is a delicious Italian antipasto. Using bresaola, an air-dried, salted beef from Sondrio and the surrounding Valtellina mountains, it takes only five minutes to make. Although they keep well in the fridge, they need to be served at room temperature to get the best flavour from the bresaola.

Serves 2
Approximately 190 calories/4g total carbs per serving

   16 thin slices bresaola
   2 tbsp olive oil
   1 tsp lemon juice
   90g/3¼ oz fresh rocket (arugula) leaves
   Generous chunk Parmesan cheese
   Freshly ground black pepper
   Bunch chives (optional)
   Lemon wedges, to serve

Place the rocket (arugula) leaves in a large bowl and dress with half the olive oil and the lemon juice. Set aside.

Lay the bresaola slices out flat on a board or clean work surface and brush over the remaining olive oil. Divide the rocket (arugula) leaves between the bresaola slices, placing a small mound in the centre of each slice, and then finely grate some of the Parmesan over each pile of rocket. Season each slice with a little of the black pepper and then roll the slices tightly around the filling. The olive oil should help to keep the rolls intact, but, if you want to be showy, you can tie each roll with a chive or secure with a tooth pick.

Transfer the rolls to a serving platter, placing them closely together for additional support, and then grate over any remaining Parmesan. Season with a generous grind of the black pepper. Serve immediately at room temperature, and with lemon wedges alongside for squeezing.

Cook's tip: As an alternative to the Parmesan, this recipe also works with small chunks of fresh Caprino goat's cheese. Don't make the rolls too far ahead of time, or the rocket will start to wilt.

CRAB WITH WASABI MAYONNAISE AND CUCUMBER SALAD

A crunchy, fresh salad bursting with flavour with a spicy hit from green wasabi mayonnaise, which is available in many fishmongers in small tubes.

Serves 2
Approximately 130 calories/7g total carbs per serving

FOR THE CUCUMBER SALAD
    ½ cucumber, peeled and thinly sliced
    ¼ small red onion, very finely sliced
    1 tbsp sour cream
    1 tsp white wine vinegar
    1 tsp milk
    ½ tsp Dijon mustard
    A few dill sprigs, finely chopped
    Sea salt and freshly ground black pepper

FOR THE CRAB
    1 tbsp light mayonnaise or Greek yoghurt
    1 tsp wasabi paste
    Fresh meat from 1 crab, in the shell
    Juice of ½ lemon
    Sea salt and freshly ground black pepper

To make the cucumber salad, place all the ingredients in a bowl and stir to combine. Season, taste and adjust the seasoning if necessary. Cover and then transfer to the fridge to allow the flavours to develop for at least 1 hour.

Just before you are ready to serve the dish, place the mayonnaise or yoghurt and the wasabi paste in a small bowl and stir to combine. Set aside.

Using a fork, fluff up the crab meat in the shell, squeeze over the lemon juice and grind over some of the black pepper. Dot the crab with the wasabi mayonnaise mixture and serve immediately, with the cucumber salad on the side.

RED PEPPER AND ANCHOVY SALAD

The Kitchen Guru and I discovered this incredibly simple salad at the exquisite Au Gré du Vin et des Saveurs Gourmandes, a tiny restaurant and wine shop with just six tables run by Patricia and Paul Sirvent. The restaurant is tucked away in the cobbled backstreets of Lille's old town. The unexpected combination of soft, silky, sweet roasted red bell peppers and the salty hit of the silvered anchovies is an amazing and super-simple combination.

Serves 2
Approximately 220 calories/12g total carbs per serving

    1 × 450g jar/3 cups roasted red (bell) peppers
    2 tbsp good olive oil, plus extra, to drizzle
    2 garlic cloves, finely sliced
    1 tbsp finely chopped flat-leaf parsley
    1 tsp red chilli flakes
    12 silver-skin anchovy fillets
    Small handful rocket (arugula) leaves (optional)
    1 tbsp crumbled soft goat's cheese (optional)
    Juice of ½ small lemon
    Freshly ground black pepper

Lay the roasted and skinned (bell) peppers out flat in a single layer on a large serving platter and drizzle with the olive oil. Scatter over the garlic, parsley and chilli flakes. Lay the anchovy fillets across the peppers in a criss-cross pattern to make a chequerboard design and drizzle sparingly with the olive oil. Cover with clingfilm (plastic wrap) and transfer to the fridge for at least 30 minutes to let the flavours develop.

Once chilled, remove from the fridge, scatter over the rocket (arugula) leaves, crumble the goat's cheese on top, dress with a little of the lemon juice and black pepper and serve.

CHICKEN SKEWERS WITH YAKITORI SAUCE

A sweet and hearty skewer set, which is a perfect starter for an Asian-inspired dinner or as simple spicy finger food.

Serves 2 (makes 6 skewers)
Approximately 600 calories/25g total carbs per serving

2 shallots, finely chopped

4 tbsp dark soy sauce

3 tbsp water

2 tbsp mirin

1 garlic clove, finely grated

1 tbsp rice wine vinegar or sake

1 tsp sugar substitute (xylitol or similar)

1 tsp finely grated fresh ginger

¼ tsp corn flour (corn starch)

2 (approx. 140g/5 oz) chicken breasts, bashed flat between 2 sheets of parchment paper and cut into 5cm/2-in squares (skinless, boneless chicken thighs also work well)

2 large green (bell) peppers, cut into 2.5cm/1-in squares (optional)

10 spring onions (scallions), white parts only, cut into 2.5cm/1-in lengths (optional)

Sea salt and freshly ground black pepper

1 tbsp sesame seeds

Place the shallots, soy sauce, water, mirin, garlic, rice wine vinegar or sake, sugar substitute, ginger and cornflour (corn starch) in a small pan and place over medium heat. Bring to a boil and cook, stirring constantly with a whisk or wooden spoon, until the mixture starts to reduce and thicken. Remove from the heat and set aside until cooled to room temperature. Once cooled, spoon one quarter of the mixture to a small bowl to use as a dipping sauce and keep the remainder to use during cooking.

Place the chicken on wooden skewers (soaking the skewers in water for 20 minutes first will prevent them from burning during cooking), ensuring not to space the chicken pieces too tightly and only using 4–5 chicken pieces per skewer. If using squares of chicken breast, run the skewer through the corners on opposite diagonals of each piece, as this creates a fold in the chicken that holds a delicious pocket of sauce during grilling (broiling). If using chicken thighs, ensure that the skewer pierces each thigh 2–3 times. If you like, you can alternate the pieces of chicken with pieces of green (bell) pepper or spring onion (scallion), or both. Season the skewers with the salt and black pepper.

Preheat the grill/broiler to medium, then place the skewers on the grill pan and brush with a little of the sauce. Place under the grill (broiler) for 10–12 minutes, basting with more of the sauce and turning regularly. The chicken should be golden and bubbling, with the sauce nicely caramelised by the heat.

Transfer the skewers to a serving plate and scatter over the sesame seeds. Serve hot with the reserved sauce alongside for dipping.

Cook's tip: A simple satay sauce made from ½ cup of crunchy peanut butter; the juice of 1 lime; 1 tbsp each of unsweetened rice wine vinegar, hot sauce (Sriracha) and dark soy sauce; 1 tsp each of sesame oil and fish sauce (nam pla); and grated ginger and garlic to taste makes a great alternative dipping sauce for both this and the beef skewers.

CHARGRILLED STEAK AND ASPARAGUS SKEWERS WITH NAM JIM JAEW SAUCE

A light simple Asian-style set of skewers with a perfect hot chilli dipping sauce.

Serves 2
Approximately 280 calories/9g total carbs per serving

    2 red and 2 green chillis, roughly chopped
    Juice of 2 limes and zest of ½ lime
    1 (2.5cm/1-in) piece fresh ginger, finely grated
    2 sprigs coriander (cilantro), leaves and stalks
    3 tbsp fish sauce
    2 tsp sugar substitute (xylitol or similar)
    ½ garlic clove, crushed
    1 (300g) prime filet steak (filet mignon), cut into 2.5cm/1-in dice
    4 fat stalks asparagus, cut into 2.5cm/1-in lengths
    Sea salt and freshly ground black pepper
    Olive oil, for drizzling

Place the chillis, lime juice and zest, ginger, coriander (cilantro), fish sauce, sugar substitute and garlic in a mortar and pestle and grind to a smooth paste. Transfer half of the mixture to a small bowl to use as a dipping sauce and keep the remainder to use during cooking.

Skewer the diced beef onto wooden skewers (soaking the skewers in water for 20 minutes first will prevent the skewers from burning during cooking), alternating each piece with a length of asparagus and only having 4–5 chicken pieces per skewer. Don't cram the ingredients too tightly together on the skewers. Season the skewers generously with the salt and black pepper and drizzle each one with a little of the olive oil.

Preheat the grill/broiler to medium, then place the skewers on the grill pan and brush with a little of the sauce. Place under the grill (broiler) for 3–4 minutes, basting with more of the sauce and turning regularly.

Once cooked, transfer the skewers to a serving plate and serve hot with the reserved sauce or the satay from the previous recipe for dipping.

WARM GOAT'S CHEESE SALAD

This is a super simple summer salad with a sharp, cheesy bite. Use a goat's cheese log that comes with a slightly yellow rind, as it will help keep the circular shape when it's grilled.

Serves 2
Approximately 450 calories/30g total carbs per serving

FOR THE DRESSING:

    2 tbsp olive oil

    1 tbsp walnut oil

    1 tbsp lemon juice

    1 tsp wholegrain mustard

FOR THE SALAD:

    1 ripe pear, peeled and chopped into 1cm/½-in cubes

    1 tbsp lemon juice

    100g/3½ oz mixed salad leaves

    4 rashers (strips) crispy fried bacon, crumbled into small pieces

    125g/4½ oz stoned black olives

    125g/4½ oz (1 small log) fresh soft goat's cheese, sliced into 1cm/½-in-thick rounds

    3 tbsp walnut or pecan pieces

    Sea salt and freshly ground black pepper

Preheat the grill (broiler) to medium and line the grill pan with foil.

Place the ingredients for the dressing in a small bowl and whisk together to combine. Set aside.

Place the pear in a bowl, add the lemon juice and cover with water.

Set aside for 5 minutes (this prevents the pear from browning).

Place the salad leaves, bacon pieces and black olives in a large bowl. Drain the pear, pat dry with kitchen paper and add to the salad leaves.

Lay the rounds of goat's cheese on the prepared grill pan and place under the grill (broiler) for 2–3 minutes, until golden and starting to bubble. Lay the cheese over the salad, then pour over the dressing and season generously with the salt and black pepper. Serve while the goat's cheese is still warm and soft.

ASIAN PEAR, PARMESAN, PARMA HAM AND WALNUT SALAD

I love the crispy, crunchy sweetness of Asian pears. They have the texture of a fresh apple but the sweetness of a ripe pear, and they complement the salty cheese and Parma ham in this recipe perfectly. Regular ripe pears are a fine substitute. They aren't for everyday eating on this regime, but this recipe is just too good to replace them with something else.

Serves 2
Approximately 200 calories/6g total carbs per serving

1 large Asian pear, cored and very thinly sliced
Juice of 1 lemon
4 thin slices Parma ham
3 tbsp walnut pieces
100g/3½ oz mixed salad leaves
Sea salt and freshly ground black pepper
Olive oil, for drizzling
1 small chunk Parmesan cheese

Place the pear in a bowl, add 1 tbsp of the lemon juice and cover with water. Set aside for 5 minutes (this prevents the pear from browning).

Place a frying pan or skillet over a medium heat and, once hot, add the Parma ham and dry-fry until it starts to wrinkle and crisp up. Transfer the ham to a sheet of kitchen roll (paper towel) to drain, add the walnut pieces to the pan and return to the heat until crisp, toasted and fragrant. Keep the walnuts moving in the pan to ensure they do not burn. Transfer the walnuts to a bowl and season with a little of the salt.

Drain the pear and pat dry with kitchen paper. Place the salad leaves in a bowl and dress with the remaining lemon juice and a drizzle of olive oil. Using a potato peeler, make thin curls of the Parmesan cheese and add them to the salad, along with the fried Parma ham slices, walnuts and slices of Asian pear. Season generously to taste, then toss everything together to combine the flavours and serve.

FRENCH OMELETTE WITH GRUYÈRE

This simplest of all dishes has provoked a great debate with the Kitchen Guru, who believes there's no such thing as a "French" omelette and that I'm a pretentious fool for even suggesting such a thing exists. It took me 30 years and the help of an elderly Thai lady who worked in the kitchen of a small Bangkok hotel to discover how to finally make this perfect dish. I'm frequently mocked for being so earnest about my obsessive omelette technique, but I reckon it's worth getting right.

Serves 1
Approximately 300 calories/5g total carbs per serving

   3 duck eggs
   1 tbsp full-fat milk
   Sea salt
   ½ tsp olive oil
   ½ tsp butter, plus extra to glaze
   1 large tbsp grated Gruyère or fontina cheese
   2 tsp Boursin cheese (optional)
   A few chive sprigs, finely chopped, to garnish
   Watercress, to serve

Crack the eggs into a bowl and whisk lightly with the milk and a generous pinch of the salt. Place a 20cm/8 inch nonstick omelette pan over the lowest possible heat and add the olive oil and butter. Once the butter has just melted but isn't foaming, add the eggs. Use one hand to agitate the pan backwards and forwards and hold a plastic fork (or a pair of chopsticks) in the other to swirl the egg mixture around the pan, mixing the curds as they start to form.

As the lumps start to come together into one mass (but while they're still soft in the centre), stop stirring and shaking the pan. Sprinkle the Gruyère cheese over the eggs, covering the half of the omelette closest to the pan handle and then add the crumbled Boursin cheese, if using. Allow the cheese to melt gently into the soft eggs as they cook, and keep the heat very low. Be very patient—too much heat will spoil the result and brown the base of the omelette.

Turn the heat off. Reverse your grip on the pan handle so the heel of your hand is closest to the pan and your fingers are on the top. Take the pan off the heat and tip it at 45 degrees towards the far end of the pan. Slip the omelette slightly down the pan so the edge hangs over the far edge of the pan. Flip the corner of the omelette closest to the handle over into the smallest fold you can achieve without breaking the underside of the omelette, and then roll it down the pan as tightly as possible. This takes a little practice.

Use a piece of kitchen paper (paper towel) to roll and shape the omelette into as tight a tube as possible. The underside of the omelette should be completely yellow with no browning at all, and it should be the shape of a huge plump cigar. Allow to stand in the cooling pan for a few seconds before slipping it onto a warm plate with the join hidden at the bottom. Rub the top gently with a knob of butter to glaze and then scatter some of the chives over the top. Sprinkle with the salt, garnish with the watercress and serve.

OMELETTE ARNOLD BENNETT

This is a surprisingly hearty dish for such simple ingredients, and it's great for weekend brunch. This recipe will make one large omelette to share or two smaller omelettes if you want to have one each.

Serves 2
Approximately 400 calories/6g total carbs per serving

  1 smoked haddock fillet (approx. 150g/4½ oz)
  1 tbsp lemon juice
  1 tbsp butter
  Sea salt and freshly ground black pepper
  3 tbsp full-fat mayonnaise
  1 tbsp single (pouring) cream (half-and-half)
  1 pinch cayenne pepper
  ½ tsp English mustard powder
  4 large eggs
  2 tbsp grated Gruyère cheese
  1 tsp chopped parsley
  50g/1¾ oz rocket (arugula) leaves, to serve
  Lemon wedges, to serve

Preheat the grill (broiler) to medium. Place the haddock in a small ovenproof dish, squeeze over the lemon juice, dot with half the butter and season with the black pepper. Place under the grill (broiler) for 4–5 minutes, until translucent and just starting to flake. Set the fish aside to cool, then flake into a small bowl. Do not turn off the grill (broiler).

Add the mayonnaise, cream, cayenne pepper and mustard powder to the bowl with the fish and stir until well combined.

Crack the eggs into a separate bowl and whisk to combine. Place a nonstick frying pan or skillet over a medium heat and add the remaining butter. Once the butter is melted and foaming, add the eggs to the pan and agitate lightly with a plastic fork (this will protect the nonstick coating of your pan) until small lumps start to form. Bring these lumps into the centre of the pan and then leave to cook without stirring for a further minute.

Spoon the fish mixture into the centre of the omelette and top with the cheese, cook for a further minute, and then transfer the pan under the grill (broiler), as close as possible, for 2–3 minutes, until the omelette is golden, bubbling and starting to puff up around the edges. Slide the omelette onto a serving plate and then slice it into quarters, transferring two of the quarters to another plate.

Scatter the parsley over the omelettes, top with the rocket (arugula) leaves and serve warm with the lemon wedges.

THAI PAPAYA SALAD

Served chilled, this is a delicious, crispy Asian salad served throughout Thailand and elsewhere. It can be served topped with any cold meat or seafood, chargrilled chilled chicken, generous lumps of white crab meat or cooked shrimp. I like to serve it on the side with a Thai green curry. My friend Weerapong said I should add a pinch of MSG (widely used as a condiment throughout Asia), but MSG isn't for me.

Serves 2
Approximately 200 calories/24g total carbs per serving

   4 spicy small red chillis, finely chopped lengthways
   Juice of 1 lemon
   3 small garlic cloves, very finely grated
   2 tsp Thai fish sauce (nam pla)
   1 tsp xylitol or other sugar replacement
   1 small firm green papaya, peeled
   ½ small carrot, finely grated
   4 small red and yellow tomatoes, quartered
   ¼ cup peanuts, toasted but with no flavourings
   1 tbsp dried shrimp (if they are available at your local Asian grocery)

Pound together the chillis, lemon juice, garlic and fish sauce in a mortar and pestle and then add the xylitol. The chillis should retain some of their shape. Set aside.

Finely shred the peeled papaya and discard the seeds. Soak the shredded papaya in a bowl of water for a minute or two. Squeeze out and discard the water and sap that comes from the papaya. Add the carrot and mix in a bowl. Add the peanuts and mix thoroughly. Add in the pounded spice mix and sprinkle the dried shrimp on top. Cover and chill for 30 minutes in the fridge before serving.

BEEF TATAKI

This recipe starts the day before you serve it. Leaving the meat in the marinade in the fridge overnight adds a sensational depth of flavour to the steak when it is served.

Serves 2
Approximately 300 calories/15g total carbs per serving

  3 red radishes, cut into fine julienne
  3 tbsp very finely chopped spring onions (scallions), white ends only
  3 tbsp dark soy sauce
  3 tbsp sake
  1 red birds-eye chilli, very finely chopped
  2 tsp (1 inch) finely grated fresh ginger
  1 garlic clove, crushed
  1 tsp lemon juice
  1 small carrot, peeled and cut into fine julienne
  ½ small white onion, finely sliced
  1 (15cm/6 inch) prime filet steak (filet mignon), cut from the tail end of the filet
  Sea salt and freshly ground black pepper
  Small bunch watercress
  Handful rocket (arugula) leaves
  Chilli oil, to drizzle

Place half the radishes, the spring onions (scallions), the soy sauce, the sake, the chilli, the ginger, the garlic and the lemon juice in a bowl and stir to combine. Reserve about a quarter of this sauce to use later, and place the remainder in a zip-lock bag with the beef. Squeeze out any air, seal the bag and gently massage to combine the flavours. Place in the fridge for up to 8 hours or overnight, turning twice to ensure the marinade is coating the meat.

Once marinated, remove the beef from the bag, discarding the marinade, and pat dry with kitchen paper (paper towels). Set a large bowl of iced water on the kitchen counter, close to where you are working.

Place a frying pan or skillet over a medium-high heat and add a drizzle of the olive oil. Once the oil is very hot, place the beef in the pan and cook for 10–20 seconds on each side, turning the meat with tongs as you work and allowing it to sit uninterrupted between turns. The outer layer of meat should be caramelised (even a little burned), while the inside should be red raw. The whole process should take 60–80 seconds or less over high heat. When the meat is seared on all sides, immediately plunge it into the bowl of iced water to stop the cooking.

Place the beef on a board and, using a very sharp knife, slice as thinly as possible. Place the beef slices on a serving platter in one thin layer, then drizzle over the reserved marinade. Scatter over the carrot and the rest of the radishes. Season generously with the salt and black pepper and serve with a watercress and rocket (arugula) salad drizzled with chilli oil.

GRILLED HALLOUMI CHEESE, FIG AND WALNUT SALAD

Chewy, salty halloumi cheese is a great flavour contrast to fat, ripe, sweet figs, and it takes less than 5 minutes to throw together.

Serves 2
Approximately 400 calories/15 total carbs per serving

    2 tbsp extra virgin olive oil, plus extra, for drizzling
    Small handful chopped fresh oregano
    1 (250g) pack of 10 × ½-in-thick slices halloumi cheese, cut into
        10 slices
    50g walnut halves
    25g pine nuts
    Sea salt and freshly ground black pepper
    2 generous handfuls baby spinach
    Juice of 1 lemon
    2 ripe figs, quartered

Place the olive oil and oregano in a small bowl and stir to combine. Lay the halloumi slices in a flat dish in one layer and pour over the oil and herb mixture, coating the cheese. Cover and set aside to marinate (not in the fridge) for 30 minutes.

Meanwhile, place a frying pan or skillet over medium heat and add the walnuts and pine nuts. Toast the nuts until just golden, keeping the pan moving to prevent them from burning. Transfer to a bowl and season with the salt and black pepper. Set aside.

Return the pan to the heat and turn up to high. Then, lay the cheese slices in the pan, retaining any marinade to use later, and cook for 2 minutes on each side, until golden brown and lightly crisp. Remove from the heat and set aside.

Place the spinach leaves in a bowl and dress with the lemon juice, a drizzle of the olive oil and any remaining oregano-infused oil from the marinade. Add the figs, cheese and walnuts and toss everything together to coat in the oil and lemon mixture. Scatter over the pine nuts and serve while the halloumi is still warm.

Cook's tip: *For an impressive finish, use a ridged griddle pan to char horizontal lines onto the cheese during cooking. If you prefer, the cheese can also be cooked under the grill (broiler).*

TUNA POKE SALAD

Poke (pronounced po-kay) is the big thing of the moment; a raw-fish dish from Hawaii, this big, bold, chunky, generous salad is bursting with fresh, lively flavours.

Serves 2
Approximately 450 calories/13g total carbs per serving

1 (250g) fillet sashimi-grade tuna, diced into 2.5cm/1-inch cubes
2 tbsp dark soy sauce
1 tbsp finely chopped onion
1 tbsp sesame oil
1 tsp finely grated fresh ginger
1 tbsp chopped unsalted macadamia or cashew nuts
½ tsp red chilli flakes
¼ head iceberg lettuce, finely shredded
½ avocado, finely diced
4 finely chopped spring onions (scallions)
1 tsp sesame seeds, to garnish
Freshly ground black pepper
Lime wedges, to serve

Place the tuna, soy sauce, onion, sesame oil, ginger, nuts and chilli flakes in a bowl and stir to combine. Cover and transfer to the fridge for at least 30 minutes to allow the flavours to develop.

When you are ready to serve the dish, divide the lettuce and avocado between two serving bowls and heap the tuna mixture generously on top. Scatter over the spring onions (scallions) and sesame seeds, grind over a generous sprinkle of the black pepper and squeeze a wedge of lime over each bowl. Serve.

MAIN COURSES

BRAISED SHORT RIB WITH GARLIC AND CELERIAC PURÉE

Short rib isn't a well-known cut of beef in the UK and it can be quite intimidating for the uninitiated, but it's a sensational cut that is full of flavour. It becomes soft and unctuous after a long, slow cooking. It's sometimes called Jacob's ladder, which is magnificently Biblical. The celeriac and garlic purée is a great substitute for mash.

Serves 2
Approximately 750 calories/25g total carbs per serving

FOR THE SHORT RIBS:
    2 tbsp beef dripping or olive oil
    2 meaty beef short ribs, weighing approximately 350g/12 oz each
    2 medium onions, halved and finely sliced
    2 sticks celery, cut into medium dice
    2 carrots, sliced into rounds
    6 garlic cloves, sliced
    2 bushy sprigs thyme
    2 tsp tomato purée (paste)
    1 dried bay leaf
    500mL/18 fl oz/generous 2 cups beef stock
    200mL/7 fl oz/scant 1 cup red wine or beer

FOR THE PURÉE:

> 1 large celeriac (celery root) bulb, peeled and cut into 5cm/2 inch pieces
>
> 6–8 garlic cloves, peeled
>
> Sea salt and freshly ground black pepper
>
> 75g/2¾ oz unsalted butter
>
> 50mL/2 fl oz double (heavy) cream
>
> Handful finely chopped parsley, to garnish

Place a cast-iron casserole dish (Dutch oven) over high heat until smoking hot. Add the beef drippings or olive oil to the dish and generously season the ribs with the salt. Add the ribs to the dish and sear on all sides until golden. Remove the ribs from the dish and set aside.

Reduce the heat to low, add the onions, celery and carrots and cook for 5–10 minutes, until starting to soften. Add the garlic, thyme, tomato purée and bay leaf and fry for another minute. Add the wine or beer and beef stock. Let the liquid bubble up and reduce a little and use a wooden spoon to deglaze the dish.

Return the ribs to the pan (they should be just over half submerged in liquid), cover and cook at a very low simmer for 2 hours, by which time the meat should be tender and falling from the bone when tested with the point of a knife. (If not, re-cover and cook for a further 30 minutes.)

When the ribs are very tender, remove them from the pan and reduce the sauce until thickened, sticky and glossy. Pour the sauce into a sieve and push through as much liquid as possible with a ladle or spoon, skim off any excess fat, and then pour the sauce back into the pan, adding the ribs. (Discard the vegetables, as they have done their work.) It is entirely up to you whether you remove the rib bones or leave them in. Keep warm, or cool and refrigerate for up to 3 days.

To make the celeriac and garlic purée, place the celeriac in a large pan and cover with cold water. Add the garlic and season generously with the salt. Bring the pan to the boil over a high heat, then reduce to a simmer and cook until the celeriac is tender. Check after 15 minutes, but it could take a little longer.

Drain the celeriac and garlic very thoroughly. Place in a food processor and blend to form a purée. Add the butter and cream and season generously with the salt and black pepper. Process again until very pale and smooth, and then check the seasoning and adjust if required.

To serve the dish, make a mound of the purée on each of the warmed plates and create a little reservoir in the top of each. Place a warm short rib on each plate, leaning it up against the purée, and then spoon some gravy over each helping, allowing the gravy to form a pond and spill out over the plate around the meat. Sprinkle with the chopped parsley and serve immediately.

LAMB KOFTA WITH ONION AND RED PEPPER AND GARLIC DIP

Lamb is my favourite meat, and this spicy, hearty recipe can be prepared the day before and refrigerated overnight (the flavours develop wonderfully), but make sure you bring the kofta to room temperature before cooking them.

Serves 2
Approximately 520 calories/27g total carbs per serving

FOR THE RED PEPPER AND GARLIC DIP:
    4 roasted and skinned jarred red (bell) peppers
    Juice of 1 lime
    3 tbsp full-fat cream cheese
    2 tbsp full-fat Greek yoghurt
    2 garlic cloves
    2 tsp finely chopped parsley
    Sea salt and freshly ground black pepper

FOR THE KOFTA:

    300g/10½ oz lean minced (ground) lamb
    1 small red onion, finely grated
    ½ red chilli, very finely chopped
    1 tbsp finely chopped mint leaves
    1 tsp finely grated fresh ginger
    1 tsp fresh thyme leaves
    1 tsp ground cumin
    1 garlic clove, crushed
    1 large onion, chopped into quarters
    1 tsp olive oil
    1 tsp butter
    Lemon wedges, to serve

To make the red pepper and garlic dip, place all of the ingredients except the parsley, salt and black pepper in a blender and blend to a smooth paste. Taste and then season accordingly. Transfer to a small bowl and garnish with the parsley. Set aside in the fridge until ready to use.

To make the kofta, place the minced (ground) lamb, red onion, chilli, mint, ginger, thyme, cumin and garlic in a large bowl and use your hands to mix everything together until well combined. Divide the mixture into 8 equal-size balls and then form each ball into a small sausage shape. Lay the kofta on a dish or plate, cover and transfer to the fridge for 1 hour. Meanwhile, soak wooden skewers in water to prevent them from burning when you are cooking the kofta.

Thread the kofta onto the skewers, placing 2–3 per skewer and separating them with an onion quarter. Set aside while you make the red pepper and garlic dip.

When you are ready to cook the kofta, warm the olive oil and butter in a frying pan or skillet over medium heat until it foams. Place the skewers in the pan and drizzle a little more oil over the onion quarters. Cook, turning occasionally, until golden brown all over and cooked through, around 12–15 minutes. The onions should also be nicely caramelised. These can also be cooked on the barbecue or under the grill (broiler) if you prefer.

In a large frying pan, warm the olive oil with a large knob of butter until it foams. Drop the kofta into the pan and drizzle a little more olive oil over the tip to cover the onions. Cook for a few minutes on each side until they turn golden and even char a little. The onions should also caramelise and be a little burned at the edges. You can also barbecue them or put them under a hot grill if you prefer.

Serve the kofta with the sauce alongside for dipping and the lemon wedges for squeezing over. This would go well with a fresh green salad as an accompaniment.

SALMON TERIYAKI

I love this very simple dish for its spicy, Asian-inspired sweetness and fresh, crunchy side salad.

Serves 2
Approximately 320 calories/8g total carbs per serving

FOR THE SALMON:
  2 × 200g/7 oz skin-on salmon fillets
  100mL/3½ fl oz/scant ½ cup light soy sauce
  50mL/2 fl oz mirin or dry sherry
  4 garlic cloves, crushed
  1 tbsp finely grated fresh ginger
  1 tbsp rice vinegar
  1 tbsp Dijon mustard
  1 tsp toasted sesame oil
  ½ tsp xylitol or other granulated sugar replacement
  Freshly ground black pepper

FOR THE SALAD:

> ½ cucumber, peeled and thinly sliced (or ribboned with a potato peeler)
>
> Sea salt and freshly ground black pepper
>
> 1 head Little Gem lettuce, leaves separated
>
> Large handful baby spinach
>
> 2 spring onions (scallions), trimmed and cut into thin, diagonal slices
>
> Handful chopped coriander (cilantro), to garnish

FOR THE SALAD DRESSING:

> ½ red chilli, finely chopped
>
> 1 garlic clove, minced
>
> 1 tbsp mirin
>
> 1 tbsp rice vinegar
>
> 1 tbsp neutral oil
>
> 1 tsp toasted sesame oil
>
> 1 tsp Dijon mustard

To prepare the salmon, place the soy sauce, mirin, garlic, ginger, rice vinegar, Dijon mustard, sesame oil and xylitol in a dish that just fits the salmon fillets and stir to combine. Place the salmon fillets in the marinade, turning to coat on all sides, and then leaving skin-side up. Cover with clingfilm (plastic wrap) and set aside to marinate for at least 30 minutes.

Meanwhile, prepare the cucumber for the salad by placing it in a colander and sprinkling with a little salt. Set aside for 30 minutes, until they have disgorged their liquid and turned a bright jade-green.

To make the salad dressing, place all the ingredients in a small jug or bowl and whisk together to combine. Set aside.

Preheat the oven to 180°C/350°F/gas mark 4. Line a baking sheet with foil and top with a sheet of parchment paper. Place the salmon fillets onto the prepared baking sheet skin-side down and spoon a little of the excess marinade over them. Season with the black pepper (the soy sauce is salty enough) and bake for 15 to 20 minutes, occasionally basting with more marinade. The fish should be firm and golden on the outside, but still tender and moist in the middle. Set aside to rest for 5 minutes whilst you finish the salad.

To assemble the salad, drain the cucumber and add it to the salad dressing. Taste and adjust the seasoning, if necessary. Toss the lettuce and spinach leaves and the spring onions (scallions) in the dressing and arrange the cucumber on top. Divide the salad between two plates and top with the salmon. Sprinkle with the chopped coriander (cilantro) and serve.

CHICKEN PAILLARD WITH ASPARAGUS, GREEN BEANS AND HERB BUTTER

This quick, tasty midweek supper dish is bursting with flavour and a satisfying crunch from the green beans. The herb butter can be made in advance and stored for up to 1 week in the fridge.

Serves 2
Approximately 480 calories/8g total carbs per serving

60g/2¼ oz unsalted butter, softened
2 garlic cloves, finely crushed
1 tbsp very finely chopped parsley
1 tbsp very finely chopped chives
1 tbsp very finely chopped tarragon
Finely grated zest of ½ lemon, plus a squeeze of lemon juice
Sea salt and freshly ground black pepper
2 bunches asparagus (about 10 medium stalks per bunch)
Olive oil
200g/7 oz fine green beans, trimmed
2 large skinless, boneless chicken breasts (about 200g/7 oz)

To make the herb butter, place the butter, garlic, finely chopped herbs and lemon zest and juice in a bowl and season with the salt and black pepper. Mix until everything is well combined with the butter and then turn out onto a large piece of clingfilm (plastic wrap) or parchment paper. Form the butter into a sausage shape and roll the clingfilm (plastic wrap) or parchment to cover, twisting the ends to seal. Transfer to the fridge or freezer to firm up until needed.

To prepare the asparagus, hold the ends of each spear between your fingers and bend until they snap. Set the tips and tender part of each stem aside and discard the thicker, woodier parts. Place a large pan of salted water over high heat and bring to a boil, then set a large bowl of ice-cold water on the countertop close to where you are working. Once the water is boiling, add the asparagus to the pan and cook for 1 minute; then, immediately remove them from the pan with a slotted spoon and plunge into the ice-cold water for a few seconds to stop the cooking (keep the pan on the heat, as you will need it to cook the beans). Dry the asparagus with kitchen paper (paper towels) and then lie flat in a shallow baking dish. Brush each spear lightly with the olive oil.

When the asparagus is blanched and cooled, use the same boiling water to cook the green beans until they are only just tender to the bite—2 to 3 minutes, and no longer. Shock them in the icy water and drain on kitchen paper (paper towels). Discard the cooking water and set aside.

To prepare the chicken, line a large chopping board with greaseproof paper and place one of the chicken breasts in the centre. Cover with another large piece of greaseproof paper and use the heel of your palm to flatten the chicken breast slightly. Now take a meat mallet, rolling pin or small, heavy frying pan and pummel the chicken breast until it is approximately 1cm/½ inch thick (but don't beat so hard that you tear holes in the meat). Set aside on a plate and repeat with the other breast.

Put 1 tbsp of water into the now-empty pan in which you blanched the vegetables and add a generous knob of herb butter. Bring this to a rapid boil, so that the water and butter emulsify. Add the green beans and toss to coat in the butter sauce. Season to taste, and then set aside and keep warm.

Place a ridged grill pan over a high heat until smoking hot. Using tongs, lay the oiled asparagus on the hot pan, season with the salt, and cook until the spears are lightly scorch-marked with stripes on one side. Turn the spears and cook until they are tender, slightly wilted and evenly striped. Depending upon the size of your pan, you may have to do this in batches. Set aside and keep warm. Return the pan to the heat to cook the chicken.

Brush the chicken very lightly with the olive oil and season with the salt and black pepper. Lay the chicken in the pan (you may have to do this in two goes) and cook until it is just cooked through and nicely striped with grill marks (about 2 minutes each side). Remove from the heat. Top each with a thick slice of herb butter and a squeeze of fresh lemon juice. Allow to rest for a few moments so the butter melts over the meat, mingles with the juices and forms a fragrant sauce.

Divide the asparagus spears between two serving plates and top each with the chicken. Serve the herby beans alongside and drizzle the buttery cooking juices over the top.

ROAST LEMON AND THYME CHICKEN THIGHS WITH CAPONATA

This indulgent, finger-licking main course has a hint of fruity sweetness in the caponata.

Serves 2
Approximately 750 calories/15g total carbs per serving

FOR THE CHICKEN:
- 4 large or 6 small bone-in, skin-on chicken thighs (about 0.75kg/1½ lb)
- 4 garlic cloves, sliced
- Juice and zest of 1 lemon (zest in strips with a peeler)
- 2 tbsp olive oil
- 2 tbsp thyme leaves, stripped from their stalks
- Sea salt and freshly ground black pepper

FOR THE CAPONATA:

- Up to 100mL/3½ fl oz/scant ½ cup good olive oil
- 1 large aubergine (eggplant), cut into 2cm/¾-in cubes, salted and left to drain in a colander for 30 minutes
- 1 large onion, finely chopped
- 1 celery heart, diced into medium cubes
- 1 large courgette (zucchini), diced into medium cubes
- 2 large ripe tomatoes, peeled, cored and diced
- 1 tsp dried oregano
- 1 square 70 percent dark chocolate (optional)
- 1 firm sweet ripe pear, peeled and diced
- 75g/2¾ oz green olives, pitted and thickly sliced
- 25g/1 oz capers in vinegar, rinsed and squeezed dry
- Red wine vinegar to taste
- Small bunch parsley, finely chopped
- Small handful toasted pine nuts
- Sea salt and freshly ground black pepper

To prepare the chicken, place the garlic, lemon juice and zest, olive oil and thyme leaves in a zip-lock bag with a generous grind of the black pepper. Place the chicken thighs in the bag, squeeze out the air and seal. Massage the marinade into the chicken until fully coated, then place in a dish and transfer to the refrigerator to marinate for at least 2 hours.

While the chicken is marinating, prepare the caponata. Rinse the salted aubergine (eggplant) cubes in cold, running water and dry thoroughly with kitchen paper (paper towels). Warm 2 tbsp of the olive oil in a deep sauté pan with a lid over medium heat and fry the aubergine (eggplant), stirring continuously, until it becomes softened and golden, around 5 minutes. Transfer the aubergine (eggplant) to a plate lined with kitchen paper (paper towels) and return the pan to the heat, adding a little more oil. Add the onion and celery to the pan and fry gently until the onion is soft and translucent but not browned, around 5 minutes. If the pan is dry, add a little more oil. Add the courgette (zucchini) and fry until starting to soften, around 2 minutes. Return the aubergine (eggplant) to the pan and then add the diced tomatoes, oregano and a generous grind of the black pepper. Stir to combine. Reduce the heat to a gentle simmer, cover the pan and leave to cook for 30–40 minutes, stirring occasionally, until all the vegetables are tender. If the sauce seems very wet at this point, remove the lid and allow to cook for a further 15 minutes, until the liquid has reduced.

If you want to add an additional background note of sweetness, you can add the dark chocolate at this stage, but opinion on this ingredient is divided—I like it, the Kitchen Guru demurs. Once you are happy with the consistency of the sauce, remove the pan from the heat and set aside to cool until almost room temperature.

Preheat the oven to 200°C/400°F/gas mark 6.

Remove the chicken from the bag. Brush off the garlic slices and lemon zest and place on a foil-lined baking tray with a lip. Pat the skin dry with kitchen paper (paper towels) and then brush with a drizzle of olive oil and sprinkle over some salt. Transfer to the oven for 25–35 minutes, until the skin is crisp and golden and the meat is cooked through to the bone. (You can make a discreet cut to check this. Chicken thigh is darker than breast and will always look a little pink.) Once cooked, rest the chicken for 10 minutes before plating up.

To serve the dish, divide the chicken between two serving plates and spoon on the caponata, either cooled to room temperature or slightly warmed, depending on your preference. There will probably be a little too much caponata, but it's wonderful cold and will taste even better the next day.

DUCK BREAST WITH RED CABBAGE

The cabbage can be made a few days in advance and works well with lots of the other recipes in this book. Make sure the duck is at room temperature before cooking, and don't forget to rest the duck breasts well after cooking.

Serves 2
Approximately 450 calories/20g total carbs per serving

½ small head red cabbage, quartered vertically, cored and sliced medium-fine

2 tbsp duck fat or olive oil

2 onions, halved and finely sliced

1 tsp mixed spice

generous grating nutmeg

250mL/9 fl oz/generous 1 cup red wine

½ medium baking apple, peeled, cored and sliced

2 dried bay leaves

2 tsp sugar substitute (xylitol or similar)

sea salt and freshly ground black pepper

red wine vinegar to taste

2 duck breast fillets (about 250g/8 oz for two)

The red cabbage can be prepared a couple of days ahead. Warm the duck fat or olive oil in a cast iron casserole (Dutch oven) and gently fry the sliced onions for 2–3 minutes, until just translucent. Add the mixed spice and nutmeg and cook, stirring continuously, until fragrant.

Add the red cabbage to the dish and toss with the spiced onion until everything is slicked with oil. Add the wine, apple, bay leaves and sugar substitute, season with the salt and stir until everything is well combined. Reduce the heat to low and leave to cook in a covered pan, stirring occasionally, for 2 hours or until the cabbage has collapsed and become tender, and the apple and onions have all but dissolved into the cabbage. Add a splash of the red wine vinegar, stir to combine and taste to see if you need more—the cabbage should taste bright and lively, but not acidic. Season to taste with the salt and black pepper and then set aside until ready to use or, if making ahead, cool to room temperature and refrigerate for up to 2 days.

Preheat the oven to 200°C/400°F/gas mark 6.

Place the duck breasts on a board and trim off any excess fibres and pieces of fat, but leave the skin intact. Using a sharp knife, lightly score the skin in a crosshatch pattern, cutting almost but not quite through the fat. This will allow the fat to render out and give lovely, crispy skin while also preventing the meat from drying out.

Place a frying pan or skillet with an ovenproof handle over medium heat until nicely hot. (Most of the cooking will occur on the skin side, so you don't want the pan to be so hot that the duck will burn.) Season the duck breasts with the salt and lay them in the pan, skin-side down. (There is no need to add any fat to the pan.) As the duck skin cooks, it will release a great deal of fat, which you shouldn't waste—periodically drain the pan into a ramekin and keep it in the fridge once cooled. It's brilliant for frying.

When the skin is nicely coloured and beginning to crisp (about 3 minutes), flip the breasts over for a moment of sizzle, then transfer the pan to the oven for no more than 5 minutes to allow the duck breasts to finish cooking. Ideally, the meat needs to be cooked to medium-rare, with a pink blush all the way through.

Remove the pan from the oven, transfer the duck to a board, cover with a piece of foil and leave to rest for 10 minutes. Use this time to reheat the red cabbage.

When the duck has rested, slice into ½cm/¼-inch slices, at a slight angle. Place generous helpings of red cabbage on two warmed serving plates and arrange the duck on top. A crisp vegetable, such as green beans, would go very well with this.

LEMON BUTTER ROAST CHICKEN WITH CELERIAC, CARROT AND CABBAGE

A delicious roast chicken dish with a rich hearty side vegetable, perfect as a low-carb alternative to a full Sunday roast.

Serves 2 generously with leftovers
Approximately 800 calories/18g total carbs per serving

  100g/1 stick soft unsalted butter

  1 lemon, zest grated and juice squeezed

  1 tbsp chopped tarragon or thyme leaves

  1 garlic clove, finely crushed (optional)

  Salt and freshly ground black pepper

  1 medium (1.5kg/3 lb 5 oz) free-range chicken, unwrapped and at room temperature (about 2 hours out of the fridge)

  2 medium sized carrots, diced

  ½ small celeriac (celery root), peeled and diced (keep the cubes in acidulated water until you need to use it)

  Olive oil

  2 rashers (strips) streaky bacon, sliced into thin strips

  Generous dash freshly grated nutmeg

  ¼ head Savoy cabbage, thinly shredded

  150mL/¾ cup single (pouring) cream (half-and-half)

For the lemon butter, cream the butter in a bowl and add the lemon zest, chopped tarragon or thyme and garlic (if using). Season with the salt and a good grind of the black pepper to taste. Beat together, add 1 tbsp of the lemon juice and beat again until well combined. Set aside.

Preheat the oven to 220°C/415°F/gas mark 6.5.

Put the chicken on a board and loosen the skin over the breast by gently working your fingers between the skin and the flesh. Go slowly, don't force it—if you do, you'll tear the skin. When you have created a deep pocket on each side of the breastbone, push 1 generous tablespoonful of the butter into each pocket. Use your fingers to push and massage the butter as far over the breast as you can. There should be a thin layer of herb-speckled butter visible through the skin. Pull the loose skin back towards the cavity, securing it with a toothpick if necessary. Rub the rest of the butter all over the chicken, inside and outside, making sure that all the skin has been covered. Season with a little more of the salt. Do not truss the chicken; leave the wings opened out. They become very crisp and are a great treat.

Pour the remaining lemon juice and 250mL of water into the roasting tray. Put the chicken into the oven for 15 minutes to get the cooking under way, then reduce to 180°C/356°F and roast until a probe registers 72°C/162°F when the thickest part of the thigh is tested (about 20 minutes per pound (0.45kg)).

About 30 minutes before the chicken is ready, start on the vegetables. Dice the carrots and celeriac into small, equal-size cubes; keep the celeriac in a small bowl of water to prevent it from turning brown. Slice bacon into small strips and fry in a skillet over medium heat in a little of the olive oil until lightly golden. Set the bacon aside on some kitchen paper to drain, but keep the fat in the frying pan. Fry the carrot and celeriac (drained and patted dry with kitchen paper [paper towels]) in the bacon fat with a knob of butter until the vegetables lose their crunch and start to wrinkle and turn brown, about 12–15 minutes.

Turn the mix occasionally and don't worry if it chars a little—it just adds to the depth of flavour. Season generously with the salt, black pepper and nutmeg. Add the cabbage to the pan. Stir well and allow the cabbage to wilt into the vegetable mix for a couple of minutes. At the last moment, (and not until the chicken is cooked and ready to eat), add a generous dash of the single cream, stir through and add back in the fried bacon. Mix thoroughly.

Remove from the oven and allow to rest for 15 minutes. While the chicken is resting, pour the cooking juices into a small pan, skim off any obvious fat and reduce the remainder to make a light, un-thickened gravy. Put the vegetable mix on a large serving plate. Carve the chicken into several pieces, mixing the dark and white meat on top of the vegetables and drizzling over the pan juices.

SALTIMBOCCA WITH SPICY STIR-FRIED BROCCOLI AND GREEN BEANS

This fresh, light supper dish works just as well with pork or turkey breast and has a deep rich sage-perfumed background note that works perfectly with the sweet, buttery Marsala wine sauce.

Serves 2
Approximately 600 calories/10g total carbs per serving

- 2 (170g/7 oz) veal, pork or turkey escalopes
- Salt and freshly ground black pepper
- 2 large (or 4 small) thin slices prosciutto di Parma
- 4 large fresh sage leaves
- 30g butter for frying, plus another 20g to finish the sauce (1 stick total)
- 3 tbsp olive oil
- 125mL/½ cup Marsala wine
- 1 large red chilli, finely chopped (or ½ tsp dried chilli flakes)
- 4 garlic cloves, crushed
- 200g/7 oz tender stem broccoli
- 200g/7 oz fine green beans
- Dash red wine vinegar
- Small handful finely chopped parsley, to garnish

Cut a large piece of greaseproof paper and use it to cover a chopping board. Cover one of the escalopes with another sheet of greaseproof paper and use a meat mallet, rolling pin or small frying pan to beat it out to approximately half a centimetre thick. Set aside on a plate and repeat with the other escalope. Place both the escalopes on the board and season very lightly with the salt and black pepper. Place 2 of the sage leaves on each escalope and cover the entire thing with the slices of prosciutto di Parma. Use 2 toothpicks on each escalope to secure the sage and ham to the meat.

Bring a saucepan of salted water to the boil and blanch the broccoli for 1 minute. Plunge them into a bowl of iced water to stop the cooking and drain very thoroughly on kitchen paper (paper towels). Repeat with the green beans, giving them 2 minutes of blanching. Put the vegetables on one side—this vegetable preparation can be done in advance and the dish will be finished/assembled after you've cooked the meat.

Place a large frying pan over a medium-high heat. Add half the butter and 1 tbsp of the olive oil and warm until sizzling. Place both escalopes in the pan, prosciutto side down, and fry for 2 minutes. Flip and cook for 1 further minute. If you are using turkey breasts, you may need a minute or two longer, but be careful, as turkey can go very dry if overcooked in this way. Remove from the pan, cover with foil and keep warm in a very low oven. Deglaze the pan with the wine, scraping up all the cooking residue with a wooden spoon. Reduce the liquid until it becomes syrupy and then swirl in the remaining butter, which will mellow the sauce and give it a lovely sheen.

Back to the vegetables. Warm the remaining olive oil in a frying pan over medium heat. Add the chilli (or chilli flakes) and garlic and stir to keep it from burning. Throw in the blanched broccoli and beans and stir-fry until they are tender but still retain some texture (about 3 to 4 minutes). Season with the salt and a generous amount of the black pepper and then add the vinegar, which will sizzle up. Toss to coat the vegetables with the vinegar.

Divide the spicy broccoli and beans between two warmed plates. Place the saltimbocca on top and spoon over the scant amount of buttery cooking juices. Sprinkle with the parsley and serve.

BLACK COD WITH MISO AND SAVOY CABBAGE

Black cod (also known as sablefish) is a rich, indulgent, super–high-protein flaky white fish that pairs perfectly with salty miso in a dish made famous by the restaurant Nobu. Actually, it's not cod at all, but if you can't find it, a regular thick cod fillet or pollock works almost as well. Make sure you allow enough time to marinate the fish before cooking, as it imparts a delicious, intense flavour to the dish.

Serves 2
Approximately 550 calories/15g total carbs per serving

Juice of 1 lime

2 tbsp mirin

2 tbsp light soy sauce

2 tbsp white miso paste (low salt if you can find it)

2 tbsp sesame oil

2 (175g/6 oz) fillets black cod (regular cod fillets also work with this recipe)

1 tbsp olive oil

1 tsp salted butter

2 rashers (strips) bacon, thinly sliced into matchsticks

1 small white onion

½ head small Savoy cabbage, very finely shredded

1 garlic clove, crushed

1 tbsp single (pouring) cream (half-and-half)

Salt and freshly ground black pepper

1 tsp pickled ginger, to serve

To make the marinade, place the lime juice, mirin, soy sauce, miso paste and sesame oil in a small bowl and whisk to combine. Pour the marinade into a zip-lock bag and add the fish. Seal the bag, squeezing out as much of the air as possible. Carefully massage the fish to ensure it's coated in the marinade and transfer to the fridge for at least 24 hours to allow the flavours to develop fully.

When you're ready to cook the fish, preheat the grill (broiler) to medium and line a baking sheet with foil. Remove the fish from the bag and lay flat on the prepared baking sheet. Place under the grill (broiler) for 8–10 minutes, turning very carefully halfway through cooking, until the fish is just cooked through and still flaky. Be careful when you turn it over, as black cod has a tendency to fall apart if handled roughly. Resist the temptation to fry this fish if you're using real black cod, as it will just fall apart in the pan.

While the fish is cooking, place the olive oil and half the butter in a frying pan or skillet over medium heat. Once melted, add the bacon to the pan and cook, stirring often, until it is cooked. Add the finely sliced onion and allow to wilt for a few moments. Raise the heat to high, add the cabbage and garlic to the pan and cover. Give the pan a good shake to coat the cabbage and onion in the pan juices. Leave to cook for 1 minute, then give the pan another shake and return to the heat for 2 minutes more, or until the cabbage has wilted. Remove the lid and stir through the remaining butter and the cream. Add a pinch of salt, a generous grind of the black pepper and remove from the heat.

To serve the dish, place a helping of the cabbage in the centre of two serving plates and top each with one piece of cod. Serve hot with a small pile of pickled ginger on the side.

Cook's tip: If you're not a fan of cabbage, black cod works just as well if it's simply half-submerged into a small bowl of warm miso soup and sprinkled with a few finely chopped spring onions (scallions).

NO-BEAN CHILLI CON CARNE WITH JALAPEÑO COLESLAW

This is the recipe that I credit with changing my eating habits. It became a staple of my diet. I would make up a batch on a Sunday, portion it up and freeze it in zip-lock bags, and then devour a portion once or twice a week. I have a supply in the freezer to this day. This is best cooked for a long time in a slow cooker for maximum flavour.

Makes 6 portions (which freeze well)
Approximately 520 calories/25g total carbs per serving

FOR THE CHILLI:

- 1 tsp olive oil
- 2 large onions, finely chopped
- 500g/1 lb 2 oz fresh minced (ground) beef
- 2 medium hot red chillis, finely chopped
- 2 garlic cloves, crushed
- 1 tsp chilli powder
- 1 tsp chipotle chilli flakes
- 1 tsp ancho chilli flakes
- 1 tsp fresh or dried oregano
- 1 tsp ground cumin
- Sea salt and freshly ground black pepper
- 1 × 400g/14 oz tin chopped tomatoes
- 1 large carrot, finely diced
- 125mL/4 fl oz/generous ½ cup red wine
- ½ tbsp tomato purée (paste)
- 500g/1 lb 2 oz beef brisket, cut into 2.5cm/1-in cubes
- 4 (1-inch) squares good-quality dark chocolate (at least 70 percent cacao)
- Juice of 1 lime
- 2 tbsp grated cheese, to serve
- 1 tbsp guacamole (store-bought or homemade), to serve

FOR THE JALAPEÑO COLESLAW:
  1 small medium hot red chilli pepper, very thinly sliced
  Juice of 1 lemon
  2 tbsp plain yoghurt or crème fraiche
  1 tbsp olive oil
  1 tbsp finely chopped coriander (cilantro)
  1 tsp ground cumin
  Dash Tabasco sauce
  ½ very ripe avocado
  ½ small head green cabbage, very finely shredded
  1 small carrot, finely grated
  1 red (bell) pepper, cut into fine julienne
  2 small jalapeño peppers, finely chopped
  4 spring onions (scallions), finely chopped
  Sea salt and freshly ground black pepper

To make the chilli, warm the olive oil in a large pan over medium heat. Once hot, add the onions and fry, stirring continuously, until soft and translucent, around 5 minutes. Raise the heat to high and then add the minced (ground) beef. Cook the beef, breaking it up with a wooden spoon as you do, until it is no longer pink, and then add the chillis, garlic, chilli powder, chilli flakes, oregano and cumin to the pan. Season with the salt and a generous grind of the black pepper. Stir until everything is well combined and then leave to cook for 3–4 minutes. Add the tomatoes, carrot, wine and tomato purée to the pan, stir to combine, and then pour the mixture into the bowl of a slow cooker set to low.

Place a frying pan or skillet over medium-high heat and add the brisket, turning until browned all over. Season with the salt and black pepper and then add to the slow cooker and stir well to ensure they are submerged in the sauce. Place a lid on the slow cooker and leave to cook for 8 hours, until the brisket is meltingly tender. If the mince releases a layer of fat, spoon it off before the end of cooking.

Two hours before the chilli is done, make the coleslaw. Place the chilli, lemon juice, yoghurt or crème fraiche, olive oil, coriander (cilantro), cumin, and Tabasco in a large bowl and stir to combine. Add the avocado, mashing it well into the mix with the back of a fork. Add the cabbage, carrot, red bell pepper and jalapeño peppers and toss to ensure that everything is coated in the yoghurt/avocado sauce. Sprinkle the spring onions (scallions) over the top, cover and transfer to the fridge for 1 hour to allow the flavours to develop.

Once the chilli is cooked, turn off the slow cooker. Place the chocolate on the surface of the chilli, allowing the chilli's heat to melt the chocolate. Stir the chocolate into the sauce, add the lime juice and stir again. Using two forks, shred most of the brisket into the sauce, leaving some of the smaller pieces intact to add texture.

If eating straightaway, divide the mixture among serving plates and serve with the coleslaw on one side and the cheese and guacamole on top of the chilli. If freezing, allow the chilli to cool, divide among six zip-lock bags and transfer to the freezer until needed. The coleslaw will keep in the fridge for 3 days.

TANDOORI CHICKEN WITH MINT YOGHURT DRESSING

My local Indian restaurant harbours too many temptations. This spicy, easy-to-make alternative is a perfect substitute, but to enjoy it at its best, the chicken does need to be marinated in the fridge overnight.

Serves 2
Approximately 550 calories/10g total carbs per serving

FOR THE MINT YOGHURT DRESSING:
   4 tbsp natural yoghurt
   1 tbsp fresh mint very finely chopped
   1 tbsp fresh lime juice
   1 tbsp very finely cubed cucumber without the skin
   1 garlic clove, finely crushed

FOR THE MARINADE:
  4 tbsp full-fat natural yoghurt
  1 tbsp lemon juice
  1 tbsp Sriracha chilli sauce
  2 tsp tbsp finely minced garlic
  1 tsp hot curry powder
  1 tsp ground ginger
  ½ tsp allspice
  ½ tsp ground cumin
  ½ tsp salt

FOR THE CHICKEN:
  2 chicken drumsticks
  2 chicken wings
  2 skinned chicken breasts
  Rocket (arugula) leaves, to serve

Whisk together all the ingredients for the mint yoghurt dressing in a small bowl, then cover and chill in the fridge until needed.

Place all the ingredients for the marinade in a large bowl and whisk until well combined. Add the chicken pieces and use your hands to ensure they are all well coated in the marinade. Cover and transfer to the fridge for at least 12 hours to let the flavours develop.

Twenty minutes before you want to cook the chicken, preheat the oven to 220°C/425°F/gas mark 7.

Place the chicken breast on top of a fine wire rack placed in a pan and cook for 20 minutes, turning halfway through, until tender and still juicy. Add the chicken drumsticks to the oven 5 minutes after the breast, and the wings 5 minutes after that. Once cooked (check the chicken with a skewer to make sure the juices run clear) turn the oven off. Leave inside the oven to rest for 10 minutes.

Serve the chicken with a rocket (arugula) salad and small bowls of the mint yoghurt dressing on the side.

THAI GREEN CURRY

This is a very simple recipe from my friend Weerapong in Thailand. He enjoys cooking so much that he's the only person I know who stays in a hotel and brings the food in for the staff to eat.

Serves 2
Approximately 600 calories/24g total carbs per serving

1 generous tbsp Thai green curry paste mix
2 (150g) chicken breasts, thinly sliced (or the same weight of boned chicken thighs cut into quarters)
200mL coconut milk
6 small (baby) eggplant (about the size of a large marble), halved
3 small red hot chillis, thinly sliced (birds-eye if you like it hot)
Small bunch Thai holy basil (regular basil sadly will not do)
4 kaffir lime leaves
1 thumb-size piece galangal or ginger, peeled and chopped into fine discs
1 tbsp fish sauce (nam pla)
Juice of ½ lemon
Dash red chilli oil (or garlic-infused olive oil if you prefer)
Pinch salt

Dry fry the green curry paste for a few minutes in a small pan with a tiny dash of the oil. Chop the chicken into fine slices and add it to the pan. Cook for about 5 minutes, until the chicken is cooked all the way through (if you are using boned chicken thighs, they will take a little while longer to cook through, but they do taste better).

Add half the coconut milk and cook over medium heat for 3 minutes. Add the remaining coconut milk, the eggplant, the chillis, the basil, the lime leaves and the galangal and cook for a further 4 minutes, until the baby eggplants are soft. Squeeze in the lemon juice, add the nam pla sauce and drizzle over the red chilli oil (or garlic-infused oil) immediately before serving.

Serve with cauliflower rice *(see page 140)* or papaya salad *(see page 105)*.

DUCK AND CELERIAC HASH WITH FRIED EGG

A rich, hearty and indulgent dish, perfect for a lazy Sunday morning brunch.

Serves 2
Approximately 900 calories/24g total carbs per serving

    4 large duck legs, skin on
    Sea salt and freshly ground black pepper
    2 tsp olive oil, plus extra for frying the eggs
    200g/7 oz duck fat
    1 onion, peeled and roughly chopped
    ½ small celeriac (celery root), peeled and finely grated
    1 tsp fresh thyme leaves
    1 knob butter
    2 tbsp fried bacon lardons or chopped bacon
    3 eggs

Preheat the oven to 100°C/200°F.

Place the duck legs on a board and season generously with the salt and black pepper. Warm 1 tbsp of the olive oil in a frying pan or skillet over a medium heat. Once hot, add the duck legs to the pan, skin-side down, and cook for 4 minutes, until golden. Flip over and cook for 2 minutes more. Place the duck legs in a roasting pan and cover with the duck fat, and then transfer to the oven and cook for 2½ hours, until most of the fat has rendered out of the duck. The duck should be dark golden and wrinkly, and the meat will easily shed off the bone. Shred the meat into a bowl and set aside.

Raise the oven temperature to 200°C/400°F/gas mark 6 and line a baking sheet with parchment paper.

Warm the remaining olive oil in a frying pan or skillet over medium heat. Add the onion and fry for 5–10 minutes, stirring continuously, until soft, translucent and just starting to turn golden. Add the celeriac and thyme and season with the salt and black pepper. Add the butter and cook for 5–6 minutes, stirring continuously, until the celeriac has started to lose its crunch. Add the duck meat and bacon and beat in one of the eggs. Stir until everything is well combined and then remove from the heat.

Spoon the mixture onto the baking sheet, making four equal-size mounds at different corners of the baking sheet. Flatten the mounds out slightly and then transfer to the oven to cook for 10 minutes. Flip carefully and cook on the other side for an additional 5–6 minutes. If they char and crisp a little around the edges, it only adds to the flavour.

While the hash is cooking, fry the remaining eggs in a little more oil according to your liking.

To serve the dish, divide the hash mix between two serving plates and top with a fried egg. Season with the salt and black pepper and serve.

BAKED SNAPPER STUFFED WITH THAI HERBS

Another inspiration from Koh Samui, Thailand, this dish, "Pla Plo," is served wrapped in a green banana leaf (replaced by kitchen foil in the West). It's a meal in itself, but it can be served with cauliflower rice (see page 140). Ask your fishmonger to clean and descale the fish, but leave the head intact.

Serves 2
Approximately 550 calories/25g total carbs per serving

FOR THE MARINADE:
  ½ (250mL) tin coconut cream
  1 small red medium hot chilli, finely chopped
  Juice and zest of 1 lime
  2 tbsp finely chopped basil (ideally Thai holy basil)
  1 tbsp finely chopped coriander (cilantro)
  1 tbsp finely grated fresh ginger
  1 garlic clove, grated
  1 tsp ground coriander seeds

FOR THE SNAPPER:

  2 medium-sized red or yellow tail snappers, cleaned and scaled

  2 stalks lemongrass

  2 kaffir lime leaves

  Chilli oil, to drizzle

  2 knobs butter

  1 lemon, sliced into quarters

  2 spring onions (scallions), finely chopped, to garnish

FOR THE DIPPING SAUCE:

  3 red birds-eye chillis, very finely chopped

  2 tbsp fish sauce

  2 tbsp lime juice

  2 garlic cloves, crushed

  1 tbsp finely chopped onion

  1 tbsp finely chopped spring onion (scallion)

  1 tsp granulated sugar replacement (xylitol)

Preheat the oven to 200°C/400°F/gas mark 6 and lay two large squares of foil on your kitchen counter.

Place the coconut cream, most of the chilli (save a little for garnish), the lime juice and zest, the basil, the coriander (cilantro), the ginger, the garlic and the ground coriander in a small bowl and stir to combine.

Place each fish onto a square of foil and stuff each cavity with half of the herb and coconut mixture. Add a stalk of lemongrass and a kaffir lime leaf to the cavity of each fish and then drizzle generously with chilli oil and dot over the butter. Top each fish with a wedge of lemon, and then bring up the sides of the foil to form a secure parcel, folding it over at the edges so that no air can escape during cooking. Transfer to the oven and bake for 35 minutes.

While the fish is baking, make the dipping sauce: place all of the ingredients in a bowl and whisk to combine. Set aside in the fridge until needed.

Remove the fish from the oven and leave to rest for 2–3 minutes before opening the parcels. Remove and discard the lemongrass stalks and lime leaves and then carefully transfer each fish to a serving plate. Serve the fish garnished with the spring onion (scallion) and the remaining finely chopped red chilli and a small bowl of the dipping sauce alongside.

PAN-FRIED PIGEON BREAST WITH WILD MUSHROOMS, CHARGRILLED ASPARAGUS AND SPINACH

This recipe is made in a single pan (with a little oven time thrown in) and comes together very quickly, making it a great option for when you want to get something showy on the table, but don't have much time to execute it! Do make sure all your ingredients are prepped and to hand before you start cooking.

Serves 2
Approximately 350 calories/8g total carbs per serving

2 knobs butter

4 pigeon breasts, skin-on

2 tbsp bacon lardons

Large handful mixed wild mushrooms

1 tsp very finely chopped fresh oregano

1 tbsp Marsala wine

1 tbsp single (pouring) cream (half-and-half)

1 tbsp olive oil

2 bunches (15–16 stalks altogether) medium-thick asparagus, woody stems removed

Sea salt and freshly ground black pepper

3 large handfuls baby leaf spinach

1 tbsp lemon juice

Preheat the oven to 180°C/350°F/gas mark 4.

Place a heavy frying pan or skillet over a medium heat and add 1 knob of the butter. Once the butter starts to foam, add the pigeon breasts to the pan, skin-side down, and leave to cook for 1 minute. Flip the pigeon breasts and cook on the other side for another minute. Then immediately transfer to a baking sheet and place in the oven for 3 minutes (and not a second longer!) Remove from the oven, cover with foil and set aside. Turn the oven off at this point, as you will need the residual heat to keep other elements of the dish warm.

Return the frying pan or skillet to the heat and add the bacon lardons, frying for a few minutes until golden and crisp. Transfer to a sheet of kitchen paper (paper towel) to soak up the grease and place in the (now cooling) oven to keep warm.

Return the pan to the heat and add the mushrooms, allowing them to cook in the fat rendered by the bacon. Add the oregano and cook until the mushrooms are juicy and tender, and then drain off the fat. With the mushrooms still in the pan, add the wine and remaining butter to the pan and cook until the liquid is reduced to a syrupy glaze. Add the cream to the pan and stir into the sauce. Pour the mushrooms and sauce into a bowl and then transfer to the oven to keep warm.

Return the pan to the heat and add the olive oil. Once the oil is hot, add the asparagus and sprinkle generously with the salt. Cook the asparagus, stirring continuously, until charred and tender, and then add the spinach and remaining butter and cook until the spinach has wilted in the pan, around 2 minutes. Remove from the heat and set aside.

To serve the dish, thinly slice the pigeon breast on the diagonal. Plate the spinach and asparagus and sprinkle over the lemon juice and a good grind of the black pepper. Spoon over the mushrooms (leaving a little sauce in the bowl) and the lardons. Lay the sliced pigeon breasts on top and drizzle over any remaining sauce.

PRAWN CURRY WITH LEMON CAULIFLOWER RICE

Sometimes, the urge for a curry is overpowering. This recipe hits the spot. Cauliflower rice is a great substitute for regular rice; it's not dissimilar to couscous and can be flavoured in the same way using any combination of Indian, Mexican or Moroccan spices. Some supermarkets now even stock bags of pre-prepared cauliflower rice in the chilled section, but it's easy to make your own.

Serves 2
Approximately 490 calories/25g total carbs per serving

   2 tsp olive oil
   1 large onion, finely chopped
   1 red chilli, very finely chopped
   1 thumb-sized piece fresh ginger, peeled and sliced into matchsticks
   1 garlic clove, crushed
   1 tsp hot curry powder
   1 tsp red chilli flakes
   200g/7 oz tinned chopped tomatoes
   1 × 160mL/5½ fl oz can coconut cream
   ½ small cauliflower, cut into florets
   Zest of ½ lemon
   ¼ tsp ground turmeric
   ¼ tsp ground cumin
   4 spring onions (scallions), finely chopped
   Sea salt and freshly ground black pepper
   Small dash dark soy sauce
   1 small knob butter
   2 large ripe tomatoes, roughly chopped
   1 (250g) pack shelled raw king prawns (jumbo shrimp)
   Juice of 1 lime
   1 tbsp chopped coriander (cilantro) leaves
   Sour cream or plain yoghurt, to serve

Warm half the oil in a large, heavy frying pan or skillet over medium heat. Once hot, add the onion, ½ the chilli, the ginger, the garlic, the curry powder and the chilli flakes and cook, stirring continuously, for 2–3 minutes, until fragrant. Add the tinned tomatoes and coconut cream to the pan, stir to combine and cook for a few minutes more. Transfer the mixture to a blender, pulse until smooth and set aside.

Place the cauliflower in a food processor and pulse to the consistency of rice. Warm the remaining oil in a clean frying pan or skillet over medium heat and then add the cauliflower. Cook, stirring continuously, for 5 minutes. Add the remaining chilli halfway through and season with the lemon zest, turmeric and cumin, but don't be tempted to add any additional liquid. At the end of 5 minutes, add the spring onions (scallions) and season well with the salt, black pepper and dark soy sauce and fluff with a fork. Keep warm until needed.

Melt the butter in a small pan over high heat and add the fresh tomatoes. As the tomatoes start to caramelise and char, add the prawns, stir for a few seconds, and then pour in the previously made tomato and coconut sauce and stir to combine. Leave to cook until the prawns are just pink (about 3 to 4 minutes) and remove from the heat, stirring in the lime juice at the last moment.

To serve the dish, place a generous mound of the cauliflower rice in the centre of each serving plate and top with the prawn curry. Garnish with a scattering of the coriander (cilantro) and serve with a generous dollop of sour cream or yoghurt on the top.

PARMESAN-GRILLED SALMON WITH GREEN BEANS, BLACK OLIVES AND FETA

In this delicious fish dish for a midweek supper, the salad of green beans and feta complements the fish perfectly and keeps well for at least a day in the fridge.

Serves 2
Approximately 700 calories/15g total carbs per serving

    3 tbsp olive oil
    1 knob butter
    2 boneless salmon fillets
    1 (120g) pack fine green beans
    2 tbsp finely grated Parmesan cheese
    1 garlic clove, finely grated
    1 tbsp sour cream
    ½ tsp Italian dried herbs
    ½ tsp Dijon mustard
    2 tsp balsamic vinegar
    10 small red cherry tomatoes, halved
    12 pitted black olives
    ½ red onion, very finely chopped
    3 tbsp mature feta cheese, crumbled
    Small handful chopped chives, to garnish
    Lemon wedges, to serve

Preheat the grill (broiler) to high and line a baking sheet with foil.

Warm 1 tbsp of the olive oil and the butter in a frying pan or skillet over a medium heat. Once hot and foaming, add the salmon, skin-side down and cook for 3–4 minutes, until the skin is crisp and golden. Check the salmon occasionally to ensure the skin is not burning, but do not agitate the pan.

Meanwhile, place the beans in a pan of boiling water and cook until just tender but retaining a little crunch, around 3 minutes. Once cooked to your liking, immediately plunge the beans into a bowl of ice-cold water to stop them from cooking any further.

Lay the salmon fillets on the prepared baking sheet and top with the grated Parmesan. Place under the grill (broiler) until the cheese is golden and bubbling, around 2 minutes. Keep warm.

Place the remaining olive oil, garlic, sour cream, Italian herbs, Dijon mustard and balsamic vinegar in a small bowl and whisk to combine. Place the cooled beans in a large bowl with the tomatoes, olives, red onion and feta cheese. Pour over the dressing and toss everything to combine.

Divide the salad between the two serving plates and top each with a salmon fillet. Sprinkle over the chives and serve with the lemon wedges alongside for squeezing over.

KAMIKAZE VODKA MARGARITA

A tribute to where it all began. Avoid commercial margarita mix. Make your own—it's awesome. No orange liquor allowed.

Serves 2
Approximately 200 calories/10g total carbs per serving

> Juice of 2 limes (squeezed lime half reserved for rimming glass and 1 lime slice reserved to garnish)
> Flaked sea salt, for rimming the glass (optional)
> Crushed ice
> 50mL/2 fl oz (2 standard shots) very cold white tequila
> 25mL/1 fl oz (1 standard shot) very cold lemon vodka
> Dash sugar-free elderflower concentrate (0-percent-sugar Fleur de Sureau by Teisseire[44] is a great sugar-free product) or 1 tsp xylitol or other sugar replacement

---

44 https://www.teisseire.com/en/global/

To prepare the glass, run half the squeezed lime around the rim of a chilled margarita glass or small tumbler and invert into a shallow bowl of sea salt, if using. Drop a handful of the crushed ice into the glass and set aside.

Quarter fill a chilled cocktail shaker with crushed ice, add the remaining ingredients, cover and shake vigorously. Strain into the prepared glass, garnish with the reserved lime slice and serve.

ACKNOWLEDGMENTS

So many people have helped me on this journey: Tracie the Kitchen Guru; my friends at work and elsewhere around the world who have listened to me bang on about this endlessly; Adam; Rhidian; Edward; Judy; Colette; Lily; Weerapong; Dr Charlotte Mendes da Costa and the good-natured and long-suffering staff at Bedford Park Surgery in West London who dealt with my sulks and stubbornness; and the persistence of the kind staff at Vision Express in Chiswick—they all helped more than they know. Their patience was matched by Dan Hurst, my wise editor, who stuck with me to help bring this book to life and Perrin Davis, whose skill and professionalism guided me over the finish line with such panache. And I'm grateful for the sage advice and confidence of my commissioning editor at Hammersmith Health Books, Georgina Bentliff, who was brave enough to add this book to her very impressive list and Dr David Levy, author of Hammersmith Health Books' *Get Tough with Type 2 Diabetes* who put me straight on some medical fundamentals, not least the difference between a sign and a symptom of a disease. Thank you so much. Mistakes or errors are entirely my own.

I'm very grateful to Professor Roy Taylor, Professor of Medicine and Metabolism, University of Newcastle, Honorary Consultant

Physician, Newcastle Acute Hospitals NHS Trust and Director of Newcastle Magnetic Resonance Centre, who gave me permission to quote his words. I'm also very grateful to Professor Mike Lean, Professor of Human Nutrition at the University of Glasgow, for allowing me to do the same. Nothing in this book comes with their approval or endorsement, and no other people or organisations referenced in the narrative have endorsed anything in this book, but Roy Taylor's and Mike Lean's work have inspired me beyond measure. I'm confident their research will change lives.

Most of all, I have been inspired by the thousands of diabetic rebels and refuseniks who have taken their destiny in their own hands and charted their own course through this malignant disease. You are in the vanguard of the revolution in the treatment of type 2 diabetes. One day your approach will be the mainstream. Until then, stay strong.

INDEX